The Grand Tetons

and the Snake River

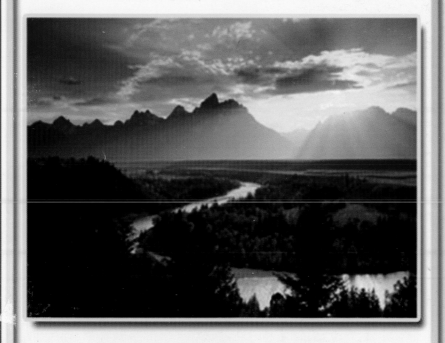

I Was Not Alone...

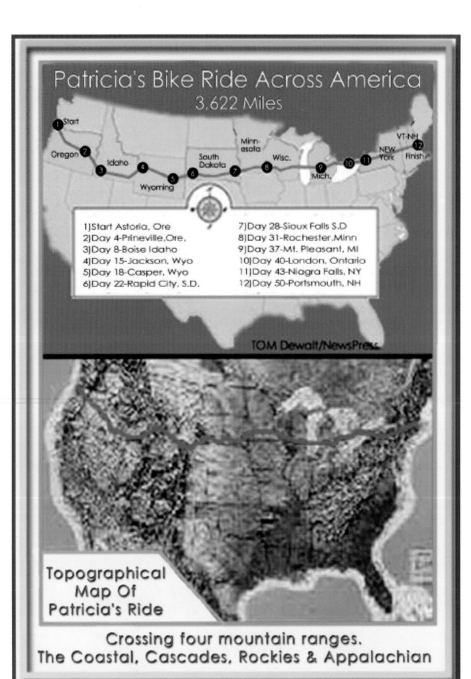

Patricia's Bike Ride Across America
3,622 Miles

Start
Oregon
Idaho
Wyoming
South Dakota
Minnesota
Wisc.
Mich.
VT-NH
NEW York
Finish

1)Start Astoria, Ore
2)Day 4-Prineville, Ore,
3)Day 8-Boise Idaho
4)Day 15-Jackson, Wyo
5)Day 18-Casper, Wyo
6)Day 22-Rapid City, S.D.
7)Day 28-Sioux Falls S.D
8)Day 31-Rochester, Minn
9)Day 37-Mt. Pleasant, MI
10)Day 40-London, Ontario
11)Day 43-Niagra Falls, NY
12)Day 50-Portsmouth, NH

TOM Dewalt/NewsPress

Topographical
Map Of
Patricia's Ride

Crossing four mountain ranges.
The Coastal, Cascades, Rockies & Appalachian

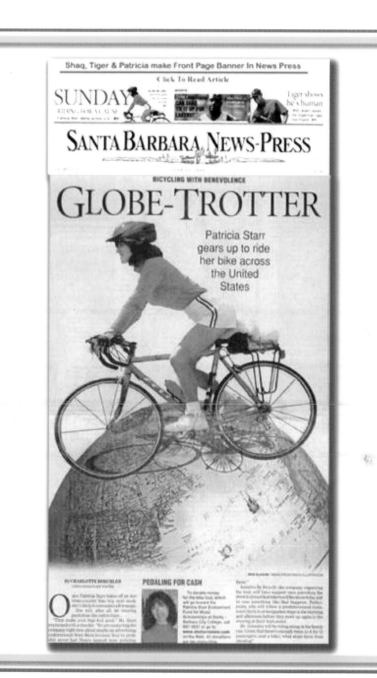

GLOBE-TROTTER

BICYCLING WITH BENEVOLENCE

Patricia Starr
gears up to ride
her bike across
the United
States

PEDALING FOR CASH

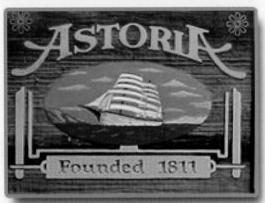

Founded 1811

Ready To Roll...

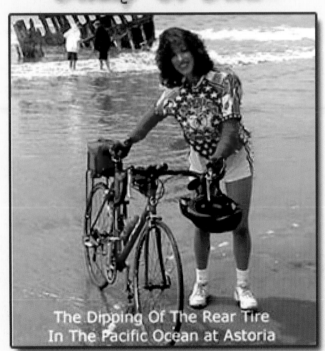

The Dipping Of The Rear Tire
In The Pacific Ocean at Astoria

Angel

on My Handlebars

By
PATRICIA STARR

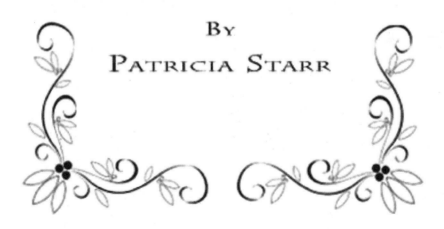

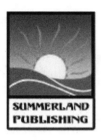

ISBN 978-0-9795444-8-4
Copyright 2009 by Patricia Starr

For more information, visit www.SummerlandPublishing.com.
Printed in the U. S. A.

Library of Congress #2009921127

Printed on Recycled Paper.

I did it again. I felt those tears slipping out from under my sunglasses. After all the long days on the road and the obstacles I had overcome – ominous electrical storms, rain, heat, wind, fatigue, hunger, a broken toe, screaming muscles, a nasty crash, panic at being lost and alone, our van being stolen – was my dream of reaching the Atlantic Ocean going to be thwarted on the last day by a broken bicycle chain?

Angel on my Handlebars is the adventures of the 50 days it took to pedal 3,622 miles across America. I was a 67-year-old woman in short shorts and Hanes Pantyhose riding a $600 bicycle with a kickstand and a fuzzy seat cover. All odds were against me. Many of the days during the ride stretched between 100-120 miles. The excitement didn't fade. It swung from angel experiences to heartbreak to excruciating pain.

Each day was a unique experience. It was ultimately an adventure story about the survival of the human spirit. Through this book, I want to inspire others to never give up. Whatever your dream happens to be, go for it.

DEDICATION

Rosemarie Fanucchi was our first "angel" as the bicycle ride came into focus. She was a well-known author and columnist, and this book is dedicated to her memory. Her support and guidance propelled us on when the negativity of others was dragging us down. She wouldn't let us give up.

I am grateful to Anne Lowenkopf for leading me into the writing world. A special thank you goes to the Carpinteria Writer's Group, the Santa Barbara Writer's Conference and author Cork Millner, my teacher for the past three years. His encouragement and guidance enabled this book to become a reality.

I also wish to acknowledge my celestial angels and my earthly angel, Gabriel, for helping me accomplish my dream of pedaling America. Gabriel has found sobriety. His sponsor, Dr. Anthony Gardiner Lowell, 61 years sober, commends him for "becoming more of a husband and friend to his wife, Patricia, and growing through the Twelve Step Program."

My goal to raise $22,000 for a perpetual $1,000 a year scholarship at Santa Barbara City College wouldn't have been possible without The Baron--radio station 1290AM, Charlotte Boeschler--Santa Barbara News Press, Barney Brantingham--Independent and John Palminteri--Key 3 TV All the young, aspiring musicians and I are so appreciative of the excellent media support.

ABOUT THE AUTHOR

A few interesting facts about Patricia Starr:

She drives a big red one-ton truck and loves to tap dance; Scott Evans, Mayor of Atlantic City, proclaimed her the "Bicycling Beauty Queen" in 2008; She pedaled 3,622 miles across America at age 67 to raise money for scholarships at Santa Barbara City College*; Governor Heineman proclaimed September 19th as Patricia Starr Day in the entire state of Nebraska; She's an inspirational speaker admired by all ages and has a "hole in one" on the Jack Nicklaus designed golf course, Pawley's Plantation, in Myrtle Beach, SC; She takes vitamins but no drugs of any kind; She plays a four-manual pipe organ; She lays tile and does concrete finishing; She wakes up happy every morning; She's a Red Hatter; To raise money for scholarships in Wahoo, NE she pedaled 1,400 miles from Wahoo to Atlantic City as Ms. Sr. Nebraska 2008** placing as 4th Runner up out of 44 contestants in Ms. Sr. America—you can read about the highs and the heartbreak in her next book, *Journey of a Lifetime*; She's a nutritionist; She and handsome husband, Gabriel, live in Santa Barbara, CA and Wahoo, NE where they are restoring their 1888 home; She has three children and a granddaughter; Purple is her favorite color; Her measurements are 37-27-37; As a concert pianist, her flying fingers dazzle audiences with Chopin Polonaises, Rhapsody in Blue and Bumble Boogie from Nashville and Branson to both ends of the country; She's hypoglycemic—a real challenge on the long bicycle rides; She loves crossword puzzles and plays trombone in an 80 piece band; She was Ms. Sr. California 2006 and 2nd Runner-up in Las Vegas; She walks two miles almost every day; She sings and directs choirs and bands and plays tennis; She survived a nasty Brown Recluse spider bite without any necrosis; She's a Delta Zeta and happily married to a "younger man"(20 years age difference); She has done high fashion, ramp and tea room modeling; She's an actress and a landscape designer and gardener; She is a photographic model; She eats peanut butter sandwiches (hold the jelly); Wahoo has honored her with an Ambassadorship; Perfume makes her sneeze; She received the Howard Hansen Award for her zeal in promoting music education; The extensive print articles across America have chronicled her activities as have Pinky Kravitz from Atlantic City, NJ to Key 3 News in Santa Barbara, CA; She grew up in a cornfield in Nebraska and is proud of it; She won an Excellence Award in Memoir at the prestigious Santa Barbara Writer's Conference; She has been honored by Mayor Marty Blum of Santa Barbara and California Governor Arnold Schwarzenegger, Diane Boxer and Pedro Nava; a 6 page chapter of the ride is included in an ESL textbook used world-wide and published by Thomson / Heinle and CNN; She hangs wallpaper; And lastly, she is an author and wants you to accompany her across America. Enjoy the adventures!

*www.SBstarrsview.com

**www.PatriciaStarrNebraska.com

En route to Astoria, Oregon

I was scared, nervous and excited. What had I gotten myself into? What made me think that I, Patricia Starr, at age 67, an untrained bicyclist, could pedal all the way across America? My dream had swept me along, but now we were actually driving to Astoria, Oregon. I never knew such a place existed before the ride preparation took over my life the past year and a half.

It took three days for the "Love Machine," our '86 van, to get us into the upper part of Oregon. Gabriel had fastened pictures of me on all four sides of the vehicle. What fun watching fellow motorists staring and waving at us.

We stopped at the Columbia River Gorge, one of the most spectacular places in the world, to give our souls a treat-- unbelievable ferns, flowers, and greenery amid multiple waterfalls-- before we became completely immersed in "pedal America."

As we passed through Portland onto the highway to the Pacific Coast, my stomach was trembling with butterflies. What about those huge logging trucks? Will there be room for me on the road? What will the other bicyclists be like? I'll be spending the next seven weeks with strangers. Will they laugh at me for being so untrained and inexperienced? What if I can't make even the first day? Will I be embarrassed? Maybe I'll have to move to another city instead of going back home to Santa Barbara.

I appeared to be so sure of myself during the preparation period; there wasn't a hint of any doubts. Now, as we got closer, they were pushing in from all sides.

From the beginning, I wanted this adventure to benefit someone else. After much searching, Gabriel and I set up a

Patricia Starr Music Scholarship at our local college-Santa Barbara City College. The fund-raising was already in motion. Would I have to give the money back if I flopped?

I was a well-prepared, confident musician when I was performing. That day, I felt as apprehensive as a kid on the first day of kindergarten. I only knew I had a goal to pedal America.

As we pulled up to the motel in Astoria and unloaded my bicycle, we were introduced to the America By Bicycle team. They were welcoming and friendly and handed out schedule details. A mechanic checked and verified that my bike was in good condition. What about me? Glad I didn't have to pass his physical. Because of my age, I previously had to send in a written note from my Santa Barbara physician stating his opinion that I was capable of long distance bicycling.

The orientation meeting was next on the schedule. As I looked at the large group of people seated in the room, I noticed 3/4ths of the bicyclists were men; and spotted only one other "older" woman. One by one, we introduced ourselves and added a line about our career "at home." After a pep talk from the leader that we would be embarking on a fabulous experience as we crossed America, we were dismissed with directions to head to the Pacific Ocean to dunk our rear tire.

Gabriel followed in the Love Machine as I pedaled the few miles. He snapped photos during my "dunking", the official act to start the ride. Tomorrow morning we would meet for a group picture before we rode off on a never-to-be-forgotten journey.

PREFACE:
ANGEL EXPERIENCE

The Grand Teton Mountains, the breasts of Mother Nature, towered in the distance. Their stark, angular lines made them look naked with only a dusting of snow for the purpose of modesty. *What a Jekyll and Hyde scene,* I thought, as my eyes darted from the grandeur of the mountains to the scruffy sagebrush dotting the desert surrounding me.

I was a 67-year-old woman in short shorts and Hanes support hose, which didn't fit the bicyclist image – neither did my $600 bicycle with its fuzzy seat cover and a kickstand.

The winds started to make mini-whirlwinds in the loose, colorless soil, the only signs of movement in the barren desert. There were no visible signs of life – people, animals or birds. I felt like I was the only one of God's creatures in the entire landscape.

As I pedaled along, I reached up to pull off my sunglasses. The first wave of panic hit when I realized they weren't even on my face; they were still in my bag. The ominous sky darkened at an alarming rate and pulled a dusky curtain over the mountain vista before me.

An uneasy feeling stirred in the pit of my stomach. There was something different about the atmosphere as the storm approached. The air was eerily calm and my breath felt like it was being sucked out of me.

Suddenly, the mini-whirlwinds turned into swirling gusts that were pulling my bicycle out from under me. For the first time in my life, I wished I weighed a hundred pounds more. I gripped my handlebars so tightly my knuckles looked like they were standing at attention under my bicycle gloves. I felt like I was stuck in a cage and going nowhere.

Rumble. Grumble. Rumble. The unmistakable sounds of a storm growled through the valley floor. I got off my bike and turned around to see the sky starting to light up. Sheets of brilliant white blanketed the blackened sky. Then a towering spike of lightning ripped down from the heavens; and moments later an enormous clap of thunder resonated through the desert. I fumbled for my phone on instinct – I knew there was no service.

I got back on my bike. With tears streaming down my face, I pedaled as fast as I could. I don't know where I thought I was going. There was not a tree, bush or building in that God-forsaken piece of America to provide even a tiny piece of shelter.

The electrical extravaganza was not only behind me; it began to encircle me. My heart raced as I pedaled along in a frenzy. I was alone. I was in the desert. I was scared. My fingers caressed the golden angel pin I always wore on my shirt collar. Please, God, help me.

Suddenly, every trace of panic and fear vanished from my body. An intense feeling of calm overtook my entire being. That must be what it feels like when you die. With a breathless silence, an angel came down and encircled my body with its wings. They were white and filmy and felt like soft gauze as they touched my skin. The weightless wings sent shivers from the top of my head under my helmet to my toes nestled in my bicycle shoes. My mind was in a hypnotic trance; I was unaware of my surroundings and no longer felt frightened. I rode in complete peace with the angel wings wrapped around me for an entire hour until my husband, Gabriel, drove up in our van and found me on the lonely road.

When I told him what had happened, he didn't believe me. He thought the desert had zapped my mind. He commented that he did notice my eyes were completely clear, although they had a translucent quality that puzzled him.

5

He said, "I don't know what happened to you; but whatever it was, something took care of you when I wasn't there."

INTRODUCTION

What *was* I doing out there alone? I had a dream to pedal 3,622 miles across America. An innocent postcard had flipped out of my registration packet for the Solvang Half Century Ride – a free catalogue of bicycle events. Why not? Into the mailbox it went.

A week later, the catalogue caught my eye in my stack of mail. It was a magnet. I couldn't put it down. There it was: I could pedal all the way across America and stay in AAA motels every night. That was it! I never wanted to sleep in a tent on the church parking lot.

Wait, how could I even dream of something so outlandish. I wasn't a bicyclist; I only rode a few charity rides a year. My longest ride was 62 miles, and I had never ridden back-to-back days.

I was a concert pianist who also sang and played the trombone. I had spent my entire career teaching, directing and performing.

Yet, the intrigue of bicycling America didn't stop. I fantasized about the wind blowing on my face and inhaling the smells as I floated down the highways. Maybe I wanted to run away from an extremely busy career. I loved my life but always seemed to be over programmed. The freedom of hopping on a bicycle every day for seven weeks was tantalizing.

But how could I tell my husband? He would really think I was nuts. He knew my bicycle spent most of its life gathering dust in the storage room.

I never did stop and think about how difficult a ride across America would be.

When my husband and daughter came home at dinnertime, they found me at the dining table working on ledger books and paying bills. My husband said, "Close your eyes, Baby, we have a surprise for you."

I obeyed, assuming they had brought something ready to eat for dinner.

"Open your eyes" they chorused.

I obliged and my eyes riveted on a new red bicycle sitting in the middle of the living room. From the black tires with the decorative red band to the black wrap handlebars, the bike was a "look alike" to my red convertible, a Classic 68 Firebird with a black ragtop.

What was happening? They couldn't possibly have been reading my mind as the day unfolded into my dream.

Gabriel, said, "I wanted you to have a new bicycle to ride the Solvang Century tomorrow. Your 25-year-old Peugeot is heavy and you haven't been training for the ride. This bike has twenty-four gears and it will be easier for you to climb the hills."

"Stunned" didn't begin to describe my feelings. I mumbled many "thank yous" and hugged Gabriel and daughter Desiree.

"It's so beautiful! I can't believe you came home with a new bicycle like bringing home a box of Kentucky Fried Chicken."

My mind was whirling. I tried not to tell them what had transpired during the day, but the mixed-up words tumbled out anyway. "I love the bike. I'm riding across America next summer. It will be perfect. I love red. We're sleeping in AAA motels."

Gabriel retorted, "What in the hell are you mumbling about? All I understood was AAA motels. The ride tomorrow starts in Solvang, 30 miles from here. Why would you be staying in a motel?"

I scurried into the kitchen to find the brochure, grabbed it and held it up for Gabriel to see. "I really want to do this. I think I can. I know I can. I wanted to ride across the country in

1976 when America was celebrating its 200th anniversary. It was impossible then; I was working full time. But I want to do it now. We don't have our automotive business anymore and can get someone to chase toilets and collect rent on our properties."

Gabriel started quizzing me, "What makes you think you can do something like that? I never see you out on your bike. Have you really gone crazy? What's for dinner? We're hungry."

I should have known it wasn't the right time to bring it up, but he had just rolled in a new red bicycle!

Family and friends echoed Gabriel's dismissal.

"Do you know how dangerous it is?"

"What makes you think you can even make one day?"

"You're out of your mind."

"Have you forgotten how old you are?"

I didn't want to hear their comments. I wanted someone to be excited for me.

Nobody was.

The dream continued. I looked at the brochure hundreds of times. Breakfasts and dinners were included – good. But what about a roommate? My husband was the only roommate I wanted. He's twenty years younger than I am and is the ultimate "Latin lover." We've never been apart more than a few days in our entire marriage.

Time was running out to reserve a spot on the 2004 calendar. Gabriel didn't even want to discuss it.

I tried. "Please talk to me. I want you to go with me. I don't want us to be apart for seven weeks."

"It's a crazy idea. What do you expect me to do? I certainly don't want to spend my summer with a bicycle seat stuck up my ass. What am I going to do every day in the van for seven weeks while you're out following some wild dream?"

I couldn't get the dream out of my mind. The new red bicycle never did go into the storage room. I started making

9

challenges for myself a few times a week to get the feel of the new bike and get comfortable with all those gears. The registration deadline was creeping up. I didn't want to miss my chance.

Pieces of the puzzle fell into place before I even knew what was happening.

Could my angel already have been at work?

Day 1:
Astoria, OR to
St. Helens, OR

69 miles

When the first gigantic logging truck, stacked high with entire tree trunks, whizzed by me, I gasped, "Oh my God." I had never felt a pulling suction like that in my life. I grabbed my handlebars so tightly my fingers froze around them, as I held on for my survival. When the truck passed, the sudden absence of the vacuum almost knocked me off my bike. Clouds of dust swirled into my face, and I inhaled the sickening odor of stinking diesel fumes.

That was my first day on the road.

On they came, one after another. The screaming power-breaking engines were incredibly loud when the behemoths were only a few feet away from my body. My mind was pleading, *Dear God, give me the strength to hang on.* My skinny little arms were trembling from trying to keep my bicycle upright.

Between trucks, my mind was spinning, *Patricia, remember, you wanted to do this.* Maybe those who said I was crazy were right.

Hang on! I heard another one rumbling up behind me.

I knew what the stretch of mountainous highway was like because we had driven it yesterday in our van as we traveled from Portland to Astoria.

It was scary when the logging trucks made the van jump as we passed on the road.

Now my miniscule body and bike felt the full force of their enormous power.

11

Yesterday, I hadn't noticed what the shoulder looked like. Now, I saw in front of me a complete bicycle path of garbage: broken glass, cans, bottles, cups, bark and pieces of wood deposited by the fast-moving trucks, hunks of tires, bolts, nails, plastic bags and a squashed squirrel.

Further down the road, I came upon a huge tree trunk that had rolled off a truck. I slammed on my brakes. The tree was lying across the shoulder and stretched into the ditch and beyond.

No one had told me they fly off the trucks in transit.

Maybe I should go home.

As I rolled into St. Helens and found our motel, I walked into the lobby on my wobbly legs. An incredible feeling surged through me.

I had survived my first day on the road.

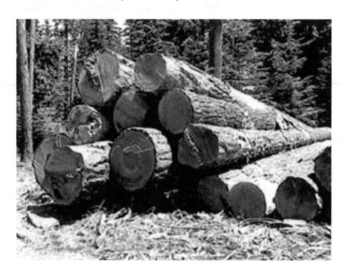

Day 2:
St. Helens, OR to
Welches, OR

74 miles

Were all the days going to be like yesterday? The first day had been a scary day. I hadn't slept well last night. Maybe I wasn't capable of "riding America." I hoped the adventure wasn't a big mistake. I had thought being in a group meant I wouldn't ever be alone.

I didn't have a pal to ride with. I noticed four or five couples together. There was a trio of doctors who had been in medical school together over twenty years ago and had reunited to pedal America. There was a father and son duo from Massachusetts. A large group of ten or twelve guys (real bicyclists) were single filing down the highway. Some groups of two's and three's were hanging together. We had a goal to pedal, so everyone took off. They all passed me. They were friendly and waved. But we all had the same objective: to get to the next destination. I was left behind in my short shorts on the bike with the fuzzy seat cover.

There were two sag wagons on the road to help us; but when they were spread over 74 miles, I rarely saw them. We signed in at a couple of sag stops; I hoped someone would miss me at the end of the day if I got lost. When we stopped, we were able to fill our water bottles from multi-gallon tanks carried in the truck that transported our suitcases. There were fruit and chips for snacking.

I didn't see Gabriel until dinner. He was trying to operate the frustrating new laptop. It wasn't working and he needed to contact Santa Barbara with daily updates. I had a phone, but it was useless in the uninhabited wilderness.

After breakfast, I had grabbed my helmet, plopped it on my head and followed the pack out the door of the restaurant. I wanted to get on the road and not be left behind. It was raining. We had been warned at breakfast to be extra careful, as the soft drizzle made the pavement extremely slippery. I fumbled to get my plastic poncho over my head.

As I put up my kickstand, I noticed no one else even had one. The other cyclists had leaned their bikes against something or laid them on the ground. Maybe I'm not so cool, but it should keep scratches off my new bike!

As I fastened my helmet strap, a nice couple noticed I was alone. The man asked, "Would you like to ride with my wife and I today?"

I happily answered, "I certainly would. Thank you for asking."

We rolled down the road single file. After a mile or so, I noticed my hands felt strange. I looked down and realized I didn't have my gloves on. Oh no, I must have left them behind in my haste to get going.

I yelled ahead, "Stop, I forgot my gloves in the restaurant."

We pulled over. Janice said, "Go back. We'll wait for you here."

I was so embarrassed, this being my first chance to make riding friends. I hurriedly pedaled back, and found the gloves by the chair where I had left them. Bicycling gloves are as necessary as underwear. They give you traction and prevent blisters.

The three of us continued toward Portland. Shortly before we were to hook up with Portland's bike path labyrinth, we saw a group of cyclists stopped by an intersection. One of the female cyclists sat on the side of the road with blood oozing from her ankle down into her sock. She was an experienced cyclist, but had gotten her cleat caught when she pulled up to stop. As she tipped over on the slippery pavement, the bicycle chain made a deep gouge in her leg.

When the sag showed up, they transported her to the ER where she got a dozen stitches. The incident knocked her out of the ride for three days. I saw how fragile we all were. That was only our second day on the road. Was I going to last for fifty days without calamities putting me on the sidelines?

Maybe I *should* quit before I get flown home in a box. But I couldn't do that either. My ride had been plastered all over our local newspapers and on TV. I was the 67-year-old "superstar" that was pedaling for a scholarship fund.

Some excellent engineering enabled us to bicycle through a large city. The bicycle path was a delight. It was a miniature freeway with a yellow stripe down the center. We soon found ourselves riding along the Columbia River looking north across the water at the state of Washington. What a change from dealing with yesterday's huge logging trucks.

Further down the bike path, we spotted some normal looking houses with attached garages. They were unique because they were built on stilts in the river. A boat could be driven into the garage instead of a car.

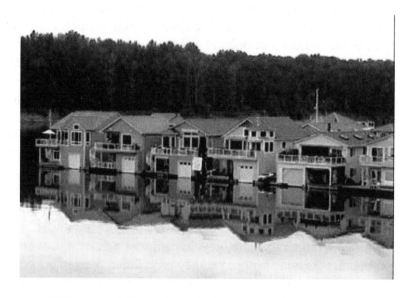

When the bike path ended, we started climbing. The road wound through a lush valley where miles of fields were planted with every vegetable imaginable. I had never seen the agricultural side of Oregon. When I previously visited my brother in Oregon, I only saw huge trees in the western half and golden fields of wheat in the eastern part. The occasional farmhouse was not large but well kept with manicured lawns.

What a peaceful ride! My new friends were aware I was not a speedy rider and were understanding of my limitations. They could have said "Goodbye" and ridden off into the distance at any time. I was so appreciative of their support.

We started some serious climbing up to the town of Welches. As we gained altitude, the trees got bigger and thicker. I struggled; I could not keep up the pace. My friends would periodically pull over and wait for me. They probably won't ask me to ride with them again.

When we pedaled into the parking lot at our destination, it looked like we were in an upscale mountain resort. The huge lodge and all the cabins were made of wood and stone. They were nestled between the trees and looked like they had been there for years.

Our room was spacious and had several windows to showcase the spectacular trees. Dinner was being served at a restaurant half a mile down the road. As we walked along the narrow road, the smell of evergreen was so intense it almost took our breath away.

After dinner, Gabriel invited the group to our cabin to view our Santa Barbara Piano Video, on which I perform seven classical piano numbers wearing clothes appropriate to the music. Between numbers, the music segues into scenes of Santa Barbara. We had spent so much time working on it and it turned into a unique video to showcase my performance and the beauty surrounding Santa Barbara.

Only one couple came. Gabriel was raring to go, but pushing the gas pedal wasn't as demanding as pedaling up mountains. Everyone else was pooped and couldn't wait to collapse in their rooms. Tomorrow would be the first big challenge as we pedaled up to ride past Mr. Hood. Would I be able to make it? I hoped my mind would quiet down, so I could get some sleep.

Day 3:
Welches, OR to
KahNeeTa, OR
66 miles

Do you have any idea what it feels like to start your day by pumping uphill for thirteen and a half miles? As I climbed and climbed, two and a half hours seemed like an eternity. I never got out of low gear.

I was feeling smug after the last two days. It had been hard work pedaling up to Welches late yesterday afternoon but I had made it. Maybe "across America" wasn't going to be so difficult after all.

I thought about one day at a time and didn't peek ahead in the brochure. As a performing musician, I have had to learn to focus. I was counting on that ability to get me to the Atlantic Ocean.

The first two days had been testing endurance but not power. My body had no bulging muscles. Some of the guys on the ride had awesome bodies. Even a few of the women were muscular.

What was going to happen to me? Climbing a serious mountain, as I pedaled around a curve, there would be another challenge directly in front. After a dozen such surprises, I was getting scared, wondering if I would be able to hold out.

The mountainsides were covered with huge, bushy fir trees. It looked like Christmas. There was no changing scenery to help propel me up the unending long grade. The road was in surprisingly good shape and the traffic was sparse.

The cold air seared my lungs. My legs were extremely tired. I couldn't push hard enough to keep the pedals going around. Not many cyclists passed me. Nobody was making any time on the mountain.

Oh-oh, here comes the ABB van. Looks like it has already picked up three people. I cannot be number four. I had to control my mind, so I didn't freak out when I saw another curve and the road going up and up.

I was freezing. The moisture and clouds were keeping the temperature down in the 40's. We were climbing to ride past the pristine, snow-capped Mt. Hood. I was pedaling in my short shorts as usual. I stopped to pull out my knee warmers, which had never been out of their pouch in Santa Barbara. When I put them on, the soft, knit fabric clung gently to my legs. At least my knees were happy. I wished there was something to keep my lungs warm.

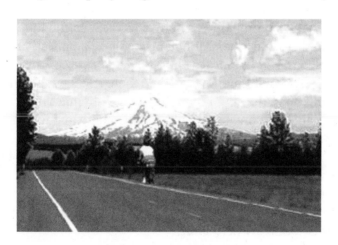

When I thought I couldn't go another inch, the sag stop appeared out of the heavy mist. I heard some of the "real cyclists" exclaiming, "WOW! What a climb." I felt a little better as that was only my third day on the road. My experience cup was empty.

The big talk at the sag was the four-mile steep descent ahead of us and how cold it would be.

John, one of the "seasoned" bicyclists, suggested, "Patricia, put on every piece of clothing tucked in your bag."

His friend Loren chimed in, "You don't know what cold feels like until you tear down that mountainside."

They were right. Brrrr, coasting down a mountain at thirty mph (I rode the brakes) was enough to freeze every bone in my body. I didn't have much padding to keep me warm. Other cyclists were flying by at incredible speeds. As I descended, I began to feel like a frozen Popsicle stick. I stopped about three/fourths of the way down to see if my body would bend. It wouldn't, so I jumped around to thaw out.

The exhilaration of the first downhill was unforgettable. A couple of the cyclists were so apprehensive, they sagged it (hitched a ride in the van). Imagine not enjoying the reward after working two and a half hours to get up there!

Even though my training was meager, the little I did was in the Santa Ynez Mountains behind Santa Barbara. One "biggie" was Gibraltar Road.

The first time I pedaled up there and saw the tiny road snaking up to the sky, I thought riding Gibraltar was impossible. I knew it was only a "hill" compared to "pedaling America."

Each time I rode into the foothills, I'd look up, pick a spot and start pedaling. Several weeks later, after conquering several goals, I went for it and got to the top.

I was so excited. I grabbed my phone and called Gabriel. "Guess where I am?"

He responded, "I have no idea."

I babbled, "I'm up on top of Gibraltar Road. I made it."

"You're where?"

"I'm at the top of the world."

"Baby, that's awesome. I now believe you are serious about the ride and that you're going to make it."

I rode Gibraltar. Practically the entire city of Santa Barbara knew what a feat that was. Public opinion (my family and friends) now had a different respect for me and started to be supportive instead of taking their usual "you're crazy" attitude.

Lance Armstrong, seven-time winner of the Tour de France, trained with his team on Gibraltar when they came to the South Coast in early spring. He likened the climb to the Pyrenees in France.

After you have climbed all the way to the top and view the entire Santa Barbara coast, it looks as it does when you are flying in. It's an incredible feeling to know your two legs got you there!

Going down Gibraltar's long, winding, steep road was frightening. I had done it at least a dozen times. The tremendous concentration that it took to descend at a fast speed tested every part of my brain and body. Lance had been faster, but I had still faced all the challenges plus the fear of flying off the mountain into space.

After a few more climbs as we pedaled past Mt. Hood, the topography changed dramatically. The earth took on a brilliant reddish hue, the trees disappeared, and I was in a desert-like Indian reservation.

It was already hot, in the 90's. My mind could hardly comprehend the freezing numbness of the morning with the body that was now boiling.

I soon learned the hills were called rollers. When the terrain was flatter, the elevations were spread over miles. Later, in places like Wisconsin and Michigan, those rollers were shortened so you were "up and down" many times within a mile.

As I began the descent into the canyon, the austere beauty of the barrenness and the vivid colors were incredible – what a contrast from the Christmas trees and snow of only a few hours ago.

It was so lonesome on the road. I had only seen a dozen cars all day. There was one tiny store, but it sold junk food. Nothing for me, so I got back on my bike and took off.

Rounding a corner, I spied one of our sag wagons sitting in the bottom of a ravine. The embarrassed staff member had gotten out to photograph the awesome beauty and forgot to set the parking brake. The van went for a ride without her, nose-first, into the deep gully.

I couldn't help her, so after sharing a few giggles, I left. She was going to have a long wait before a tow truck could make it out there. At least she had two-way radio to communicate with the world—not like my cell phone that had no call service in the wilderness.

I discovered at the end of the day that Gabriel had been her Good Samaritan. When he came along, he quickly saw she was in an undesirable situation. He pulled out his towing chain and went to work to get her van out of the gully. He was successful and the grateful employee gleefully called and cancelled the tow truck. She knew she still had to cope with the "How could you be so stupid?" remarks, but at least Gabriel's tow was free!

The evening's destination, KahNeeTa Resort, was an angular structure perched high upon the side of a mountain. Oh no! That meant another mountain to climb, if I wanted a bed to sleep in.

We had been told about the mile-long climb up to the resort. When I reached the bottom of the driveway, my body was on empty. As I looked up the hill to that beautiful resort, it seemed to be ten miles up instead of one. I was out of gas!

Gabriel and the Love Machine were already at the top. He could see the little speck, me, starting to climb and then after a few feet, stop. I took a drink of water, but I had no food left.

My phone rang! Surprise! It worked!

It was Gabriel. "Come on Baby, you can do it."

I must have tried a dozen times and had barely started up that long, long hill. I had already climbed thirteen and a half miles up to Mt. Hood, three shorter climbs, and countless hills, working my way into the cinnamon colored canyon.

With my body fuel at zero, no matter how many times Gabriel called to encourage me, I could only go a few feet further. I was getting nowhere, and my flesh was steaming hot as the temperature spiked in the late afternoon.

Gabriel realized he would have to come down to meet me, not to give me a ride (he knew I wouldn't accept that), but to bring me food. I sat beside the van soaking up the shade it made and drinking cold water from a bottle Gabriel pulled out of our cooler. The water on my bike had been as hot as I was, over a hundred degrees.

The previous night, Gabriel and I had discussed how we were going to handle my hypoglycemia. I felt like I was starving to death. We had eaten spaghetti dinners the past few nights. My body never did what was normal. It used the energy from carbs in a flash and then my fuel reserves dropped quickly. I was ravenous before I went to bed at night, only a few hours after eating dinner.

That day, Gabriel had gone shopping and filled our cooler with yogurt, soymilk, bagels, cheese and crackers. A brilliant choice, that one decision was going to be the key to get me across America.

Earlier, as we prepared for my adventure, he had said many times he didn't know what his role would be that summer. He was already handling the publicity, communicating with TV, radio stations, newspapers, and setting up interviews for local coverage along the way. He needed to devote mornings to media things and getting pictures and stories back to Santa Barbara. Our computer-friend-guru, Tom, up-dated the website every day to keep my supporters involved.

Now, Gabriel assumed another role: to keep me in working condition with plenty of fuel. He would have to catch me somewhere along the route, before I sank physically and mentally from lack of food. There were no corner mini-marts to stop and shop in the desolation.

We usually had a substantial breakfast. I left the dining room with the three back pockets on my bicycle shirt stuffed with peanuts, a banana and a couple of pancakes. (Don't worry, no mess; I'm the one who can't eat syrup!) The energy bars that other cyclists ate were "no-no's" for me because of their sugar and caffeine, two things my body doesn't tolerate.

After the spot of shade and the cold water lowered my body temperature, Gabriel pulled out the contents of the cooler and watched me devour the food.

Fifteen minutes later, I said, "OK, here I go."

I did have to stop a few times to "refuel" my legs—hop off the bike and relax a minute, then back on to ride a little further.

Slowly, I conquered the last physical challenge of the day. I didn't know a mental one was brewing.

As I struggled up the hill, other cyclists were watching me from their balconies.

"Think she'll make it?"

"Nope."

"What do you want to bet, she'll hitch a ride."

They were still curious about me, the bicycle broad that didn't fit the "mold." They watched me struggling; but as I got closer to the casino, they started clapping for me. They saw for the first time how determined I was. They knew I could have hopped in the van at any time or pushed my bike up the steep incline. That was an exhilarating moment for me – approval from some "real cyclists."

It boggled my mind to be in such a beautiful place in the middle of the God-forsaken desert. The super modern architectural structure housed the unmistakable smell and clanging jangle of a casino.

After the bizarre cold and heat changes from 40 to 100 degrees within a few hours, my befuddled mind was spinning. Were we in Las Vegas? There were a few gamblers around but not a big crowd. Most of my fellow cyclists disappeared into their rooms. They, like me, were not interested in a smoky casino.

The exception was Gabriel. He finally showed up at 2:30 a.m. He had done a little gambling and a lot of drinking. I didn't know how I was going to survive those seven weeks. The golden angel pin on my shoulder (a gift from Gabriel) had a full time job. Not only was my physical body going to be tested in every possible way, my mental state would be frazzled by Gabriel's alcoholism if it went completely out of control. He had started drinking occasionally a few years ago after being sober for fifteen.

As our plans for the ride grew over the last year and a half, so did his drinking. We were a team in everything but alcohol. We had survived Gabriel's nasty divorce and his family not speaking to him for five years because of lies spread by his ex. It was my turn; I needed his support. Pedaling across America was the biggest adventure we'd been through in our eight years together.

I loved him, I worried about him, and I couldn't sleep when he was out drinking. He was not a physically abusive drunk, only verbally—he wouldn't stop talking and arguing. At home I could disappear into another room; but in our hotel room, there was nowhere to go.

My alarm was set for 4:30 a.m. How was I going to make it to Prineville, our next destination, after an almost sleepless night?

I only wanted a bed in a nice air-conditioned room for some sweet dreams. Mt. Hood hadn't conquered me but maybe alcohol would.

25

Day 4:
KahNeeTa, OR to Prineville, OR

61 miles

While climbing out of the cinnamon colored canyon, I felt like I was on a Western movie set. I was so into the scene that I missed a turn and cycled four extra miles. Because of the brevity of last night's sleep, I was extremely tired. When I got back on track, honey-colored grazing land with sheep and goats rolled on forever. Remembering all the ups and down of yesterday, both the topography and the temperature, the day was all in the "normal" range and a welcome change for those of us on two wheels.

That day was the perfect time to talk about one of the realities of the road: saddle sores. An indelicate subject, perhaps, but the problems were far reaching. Many hours in the bicycle saddle with friction of the seat against skin caused the lesions. The next step was infection due to warmth and moisture.

Some contenders in the Tour de France have had to withdraw from the competition because of the unmentionables, which were also a subject of discussion among our group of cyclists. One gentleman had already headed home because of the malady. Several others had spent time in the sags because of the problem.

Well-meaning fellow cyclists had tried to scare me into purchasing bicycle shorts with the chamois pad insert. They said I must have proper attire to survive the cross-country ride.

I was perfectly happy with my short shorts and Hanes support hose. I was of the belief that air and circulation were the best protection against the extremely painful sores.

Some of the riders were advised not to sit on anyone's furniture. Their bicycle shorts, filled with "goo" (for supposed protection) might leave grease spots on said furniture. Yuck!

I had decided to take my chances and stick with my short shorts!

Day 5:
Prineville, OR to John Day, OR

117 miles

It took five more minutes of Gabriel's pleading before I agreed to try one more mile in the blistering heat. I was the only bicyclist left on the road. Common sense would be to get in the van, turn the cold air up and be thankful to ride the last thirty miles.

But I had a dream to pedal.

117 miles: that long day had caught my attention the first time I looked ahead at our itinerary before we left Santa Barbara. A century, a hundred mile ride, was something I had never attempted; plus, I had to pedal seventeen additional miles. It was in Oregon's upper desert. It must be flat. How else could we handle so many miles early in the trip? How wrong I was.

Now I understood the phrase that the mileage "is what it is" because there was no place in between that could accommodate us for the night.

We had several meetings during the past few days. We would be pedaling into a blistering hot, dry desert. I was already apprehensive. The leader and the medical director spent an entire session talking about dehydration and its life threatening effects.

When body chemistry gets out of balance, drinking only water will not correct the imbalance. That can lead to other systems in the body shutting down and the need for emergency hospitalization.

I had never tasted a sip of Gatorade – the magical drink to keep your electrolytes in balance. Now, I learned, it upsets some stomachs or causes diarrhea; not anything to look forward to when you have 117 miles to pedal. I came out of the meetings in a quandary, but also deciding I wasn't going to try Gatorade! I'd have to handle the salt/water balance some other way. I took to munching salted chips, something I rarely ate.

When we started our day, the road wound along rippling streams in a forested area. I had no clue what was to transpire for the rest of the day.

Gabriel didn't know that he would be crucial to my survival on many of the extremely difficult days. He was still struggling with computer issues and trying to get the laptop to work.

We climbed in the early hours. The cool morning weather ended about ten o'clock as the terrain flattened out. The barren landscape was rapidly heating up. By eleven o'clock it was already baking hot. I was alone, as usual, and getting nervous about the day.

As I pedaled up the second big climb, my body was burning and my energy level was completely zapped. There was a rest stop coming up in a few miles; but every pump on the pedals was starting to feel like my last. I tried to call Gabriel, but there was no communication.

When I finally dragged into the rest stop, a decision had been made in which I actually had no say: the sag wagon was picking up the last five riders. I was one of them. In one way, it was a blessed relief, because I had no choice. On the other hand, I was adamant about staying out of the sag.

I could have refused, but not in good conscience; one of the younger riders was already into the first stage of heat stroke. All of us had to be grouped closer, in the event that one of the two wagons might have to rush the stricken teenager to the hospital.

What could I say? When someone was dangerously ill, I couldn't be selfish and uncooperative because I wanted to keep pedaling. Into the wagon I went with four other cyclists.

I was determined to make up the extra miles some other day. In fact, I already had four of them from daydreaming and being lost at KahNeeTa yesterday. I was not going to arrive in Portsmouth, New Hampshire having pedaled less than 3,622 miles.

We got a ride up the rest of the mountainside, which consisted of seven miles of switchbacks. The climb would have taken a long time, especially in the boiling heat, and spread the group out even more.

When I got out of the air-conditioned sag, I almost fainted. I had stepped into a blast furnace. As I got back on my bike, the temp was still soaring. It was over 100 degrees.

After an hour of struggling in the heat, I thought I was going to be the next one en route to the hospital. What *was* I doing alone in such a place of desolation? I usually considered myself reasonably sane, maybe a bit "out of the box." But I was beginning to wonder…

By the tenth mile, I was so hot my face matched my red metal bicycle frame. There was one little bush by the side of the road, and that was it. Visibility stretched to the horizon for miles and miles in the barren landscape.

I pulled my bike under the bush. I stared ahead and knew that without even a promise of shade, I would curl up and die if I had a flat tire or any other problem.

Memories of Nebraska came back. They used to say it was "so hot you could fry an egg on the sidewalk." You could have fried an egg on my helmet. It burned my fingers to touch it.

When the last bicycle went past me, I yelled, "Send the sag for me if you see it anywhere. I can't go out into that furnace alone."

After waiting about forty minutes and getting hotter and hotter, I heard a van approaching. I hadn't seen another vehicle for hours. My heart pounded. Getting into the sag wagon would mean failure to conquer all the elements. How could I say "I'm a quitter" to everyone back home? I didn't even know what those words meant; but I was hot, scared and alone.

When I looked up, it wasn't a red or white sag. It was Gabriel in our beautiful blue "Love Machine." He had no idea that I was in trouble, but had a hunch he should be looking for me.

His sudden appearance, when I was ready to collapse from the heat, must have been the work of my angel.

It was after one o'clock, and I still had 71 miles to go. How could I do it? Stretching out ahead was desert and more desert, and I was already way behind the other riders.

Gabriel soaked my clothes with water from a spray bottle, fed me and gave me cool water to drink. Now I could face the endless desert, because I was no longer alone. We stopped every mile or two, so he could spray me again. As soon as I rode 100 yards, my clothes were completely dry.

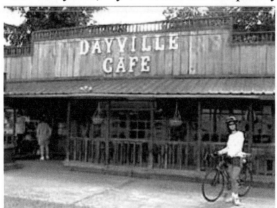

It seemed like an eternity, but we made the next forty miles, stop and go, to the last rest stop. It was a quaint Mom and Pop style restaurant. It was after 4:00 pm, and everyone else had come and gone. The owners said half a dozen hot, tired cyclists couldn't take the heat any more and opted to hop in the cool sag for the last 30 miles.

I collapsed in our booth inside the restaurant with the fan blowing on me. I mumbled, "I need food and I can't go any further. I cannot ride thirty more miles in this heat. Don't even talk to me about it. I'm quitting for the day."

Gabriel pleaded, "At least think about it. I didn't follow you all the way out here for you to decide to quit."

"I'm so hot I don't care anymore."

"I've known you for fifteen years and never heard those words come out of your mouth. I really don't want to hear them this afternoon either. You are not a quitter. At least give it a try."

"But I'm so hot and tired."

Gabriel fired back, "I'm really getting upset with you. You're the one who wanted to do this when everyone else, including me, thought you were crazy. What did you expect? That this was going to be easy? Am I going to have to call the radio station, the newspapers and your supporters and tell them you're quitting on the fifth day of the ride? What about all the music scholarships you were pedaling for? Was all that a bunch of bull? I'm mad." Gabriel slammed his fist down on the table so hard my lifeless body quivered. He barked, "I don't even feel like eating my lunch."

"You have no idea what I went through before you found me hiding under the last bush," I whined. You know how I struggled all afternoon. I am so strung out, I probably can't even get my body out of this booth."

After a really good roast beef sandwich and two cold glasses of lemonade, Gabriel tried again. "Come on, Baby, you can do it. I know you can."

My body was finally beginning to cool down, and the late lunch started to pick up my blood sugar. I said, "OK, I will try one more mile. The horrendous heat has ground me down; I feel like I'm a blob of putty."

Gabriel assured me, "You won't be alone. I'll keep you in my mirror."

Slowly, I conquered the first mile. One by one the next few miles dropped away. Gabriel was getting excited. Like the boxing fan that he is, he said I was the fighter down on the mat, getting the final count, and suddenly had a spark of life still in me. When we stopped for water and a spray, he gave me the biggest hug. "Baby, you pulled off a miracle. You were so far gone in the restaurant, even I was getting scared you might not make it."

Although it was late afternoon, the blistering sun was so hot on my body, it felt like it was being concentrated through a magnifying glass. I've never felt "burning sun" like that; the heat actually hurt my skin.

Then a miracle happened. My helmet started cooling off; the sun had started hiding under some clouds fluffing up in the sky. Was my angel at work?

Gabriel said, "I'm beginning to believe there is something out there taking care of you."

The sun would blister for a while and then a few more wispy clouds would give me some relief. It didn't help my tired legs, but at least I could keep pushing. We didn't have to stop every mile, as we had before.

After we had gone thirteen miles, something momentous happened: I crossed the invisible line that signaled my first century. Who would have thought I could pedal a hundred miles, and under those conditions? I jumped off my bike and threw my arms up in the air with a few war whoops and kisses sent up into the hot sky. After that milestone, it was one slow pedal at a time. I was not going to give up, and Gabriel egged me on every time we stopped.

That moment would not have happened if Gabriel hadn't come along when he did. He encouraged me to do something I thought was impossible. Now, I knew I could survive any challenge that would be dished out in the next six weeks.

We didn't get to the John Day stop until 7:30 p.m. as the sun was starting to settle down on the horizon. I had been on my bike since 6:15 in the morning. The rest of the cyclists had finished dinner. I think they got a taste of what makes Patricia tick: a husband who will not let her give up and her own stamina.

Gabriel was ecstatic. "Baby, you amazed me. You didn't let the desert defeat you."

I knew they had been talking about me, the old broad who showed up with a handsome "boy" to take care of her. I had probably been pegged as a "princess wannabe" who was going to quickly get knocked out of her dream. They all had a rough day, too, and were astonished I had survived. After that day, I could feel they were pulling for me. I had earned some more "biker respect."

Certainly a day to remember: my first century!

Day 6:
John Day, OR to
Baker City, OR

81 miles

The overwhelming loneliness and desolation – I was
scared out there by myself. I felt so vulnerable. There wasn't
anyone, anywhere. I had been alone for hours. Tears were
running down my cheeks. I really needed to see another
human being as I pedaled along in Oregon's desert wasteland.

It was unbelievable; I was alive after yesterday's
marathon, 117 miles. Determination would also get me through
another day.

None of the bicyclists I had spoken to before leaving
home had mentioned dealing with *loneliness and isolation* as I
pedaled across some of the most desolate sections of the United
States. They were all guys, so that may explain why.

The America by Bicycle group consisted of ten women
and thirty-eight men. The men can't know what it feels like for
a woman to be alone and feeling helpless.

Three of the women were fast riders and always
burning up the road together. Three others rode with the three
docs on the tour. They, too, were good cyclists.

Two women had husbands they rode with occasionally.
Their husbands were faster than they, but if the situation
warranted it, they did ride together.

One lady was slow, like me, but we had different riding
patterns. She spent a lot of time in the sag wagon when the
going got tough. My goal was to pedal every inch.

That left me riding alone. I was not sorry or sad. I
enjoyed being able to stop and get a drink when I wished. I

35

loved to hop off my bike and stretch my legs when the going was really tough. When I was climbing, I stopped and set my bike on its kickstand and turned around to see where I came from. The vistas were magnificent.

Many of the cyclists were goal oriented. They wanted to "get there" and their objective was seeing how fast they could accomplish it. They rode with their heads down. I'm not interested in spending my day looking only at the road and the butt of the person in front of me.

My joy was in the journey. I wanted to experience everything, as long as I got there in time for dinner leftovers and could lay my head on a soft pillow in a cool hotel room.

There was no one else like me. It wasn't that they didn't "like me." I was friendly with everyone, but cycling habits differ for each person.

Gabriel came along in the afternoons, sometimes early, sometimes late. He could not drive along with me at my pokey speed of eight to ten miles per hour or less, so he was along the route somewhere, anywhere from one to fifty miles away.

When the heat was unbearable and the climbs were tremendously steep, he tried to stay closer. He sprayed my clothes with water and gave me something cool to drink. When the stretches were long, he would hang back and read, talk on the phone or go sightseeing and then catch up to me. I was alone for many hours after the rest of the cyclists passed me by.

I could have spooked myself right out of the ride. A frightening memory kept trying to creep back into my thoughts about an incident that happened "in my own back yard."

My stalker.

While I pedaled along the California coast one sunny afternoon, I stopped my bike to get a drink. An old maroon van with silver horizontal stripes pulled up and parked. The random width striping was a popular paint look from the 80's.

The van had a lot of rust on it and some holes that looked like bullet holes. There were old broken Venetian blinds on the windows that swung freely.

Something was starting to make me feel extremely uncomfortable.

Then I got a glimpse of the driver: dark skinned, lots of curly, black hair and a bushy beard. His large body looked like a big hairy bear crammed into the driver's seat.

When I absorbed the whole picture, chills started running up and down my spine. I cooled off in a hurry although I had been hot from riding on the summer day.

I was careful to not make eye contact with him. I got on my bike and started pedaling back up the beach. The whole scene gave me the creeps. I rode north until I found our van and hung out there waiting for Gabriel to get out of the water. Somehow, cycling wasn't as much fun that day.

The summer of 2003, a year before the bicycle ride, Gabriel had resumed a teen-age love, surfing. We lived in one of the most beautiful coastal areas in the world and there were a few good surfing spots. Going south out of Santa Barbara toward Ventura, Scenic Highway 1 had a ten-mile leg that ran along the beach after it broke off of Highway 101.

It was a haven for campers. For a daily fee, you could enjoy the beach and stay overnight. Or you could park your car for free, sneak across the highway between a blur of speeding cars and jump into the ocean.

Twenty years had passed since Gabriel had been on a board. He had a really rough day; ate a lot of sand, and was moaning continuously about how much his body hurt. He had gotten slammed on the bottom a few times and decided it wasn't much fun anymore.

Somehow, the lure of surfing, or maybe the desire to prove his forty plus body could do it, prompted him to try again. He had some experiences that were more positive so he was enticed to go back.

37

Along the ten-mile stretch, cyclists shared the road and parking areas with the cars and campers. The last mile and a half was a totally isolated bike path leading to Emma Wood State Beach Park north of Ventura.

The bicycle path had an elevated freeway on one side, so it was like riding on a shelf. On the other side were railroad tracks and bushy-type brush. Then the terrain dropped to the beach with the ocean beyond. Sometimes there were other cyclists on the stretch; oftentimes no one was there. There was no escape route.

The ride across America was a year away, but I knew I had to get some miles in. Sometimes when Gabriel went surfing, I would put my bike in the van and tag along. I would start riding as soon as the highway leg began, and then Gabriel would continue driving until he found the spot he liked to surf.

As I pedaled south, I could see the parked van and would know he was in the water somewhere in the area. I rode past all the campers and onto the real bike path; went into Emma Wood Park, turned around and rode back to the spot where Highway 1 started. That was a twenty-mile loop. After a while I started putting in a few double loops to get forty miles of road time. By then, Gabriel had enough of the waves. We both got to do what we wanted, as he doesn't like to bike and I can't swim.

What a perfect place to train. It was flat so I could cruise without any effort; and riding along the ocean was heavenly. The smells, the sounds, and the beauty of the ocean and sky always validated that we really did live in a paradise.

A parking lot was adjacent to the bike path leading to Emma Wood Park. Cars were there; people were friendly and we often said, "Hi." It had been a family camping area for years.

The next time Gabriel went to surf, I tagged along. I hadn't mentioned my apprehension concerning "hairy bear." I

38

told myself I would not let a rusted out van and one creepy guy spoil my day.

As I pedaled south, the old maroon van passed by me. *Oh no, not him again. Well, he has a right to the road, too.* I kept going. After a few minutes, I noticed he was coming down the road towards me. He had made a U-turn in the middle of the road! I was careful to not make eye contact. Silly me, I forgot I had my sunglasses on. I was acting on instinct. *Maybe he'll go away.*

Even though I was 67 years old, I still looked pretty hot in my short shorts and Hanes support hose. Was I going to have to deal with "being a target" on my ride across America?

I rode past the parking lot by the bike path and on down to Emma Wood Park where I turned around. The entire area was deserted. My heart was thumping like crazy, and I was disgusted at myself for showing signs of fear.

As I came off the bike path, the old maroon van with the hairy bear at the wheel was waiting in the parking lot like a big vulture. I kept going north. I wanted to get back to the safety of my husband and our van.

The maroon van started following me. The driver got extremely close. If he moved over a few more inches, he could knock me off my bike; open the van doors and shove me in. Because I was riding north, all the ocean activity was across the road on the other side of the van. No one would have been able to see what was happening.

Fear now overcame me. He drove slowly ahead of me; traveled about a quarter of a mile, turned around and stopped in the bike path facing me.

I didn't want to approach him, so I quickly crossed the road, turned around and started riding away. The whole scene happened again. I knew he was playing with me. That was one of the sections along the ten-mile stretch where there were neither campers nor houses.

I was panicked. I had a phone, but Gabriel was in the ocean. I knew his cell was in the van.

The hairy bear did that FOUR times. He could probably see my heart pounding through my red turtleneck when he pulled his van around to face me. When he went up to turn around for the fifth time, there was a curve in the road; I was briefly out of his sight.

I jumped off my bike and hurriedly pushed it across the road. I squeezed my bike and body behind one of the larger cars parked there. Of course, if he couldn't see me, I couldn't see him either. I crouched behind the car for about fifteen minutes.

My heart was still jumping up and down. I had no idea if he was up north where our van and my husband were, or if he was down south waiting by the entrance to Emma Wood Park. There were no people around. They park their cars there and scurry down to the beach.

I had to make a decision and go for it. My guardian angel must have been on duty. I pulled my bike out from behind the big car, got on and started racing north. I only wanted to get back to Gabriel. I usually was not a fast rider, but I swear to God, I rode like Lance Armstrong for the seven miles back to our van.

I saw Gabriel getting out of the water and coming to the van. I blurted, "I'm so wigged out. There was a creepy guy in an old van with bullet holes in it that was following me and playing games with me and keeping me from riding in my bike path."

"Hey, slow down a minute. I can't even understand you. You're stuttering and as pale as a ghost."

"Baby, I'm freaked out. There wasn't anyone else around, and I was so scared."

"OK. Get on your bike; ride south; and pretend like nothing has happened. I'll follow you and not let you out of my sight. I have my camera in my hand. Raise your right hand if you see him again."

My mind was still paralyzed from fear, but now I was not alone. When I rounded the corner before the parking lot by the entrance to Emma Wood Park, I saw the maroon van with the rusty bullet holes and the hairy bear crammed into the driver's seat.

I raised my right arm, our pre-arranged signal. I rode slowly by the van and caught a glimpse of the driver's face; enough to see that he was snoozing! Gabriel pulled up behind the van; took pictures of the license plate; slowly drove alongside and snapped a photo of the man.

I quickly turned around, headed north, and passed the hairy bear again. Gabriel followed, and as soon as he could pull over, we threw my bike in the van and took off.

I was freaked out. I had nightmares about the guy for weeks.

We had identifying evidence, but what should we do with it? My conscience told me to notify the authorities. Because it had been a family oriented area for so long, parents were lax concerning the whereabouts of their kids. They thought it was a safe area. If the guy was harassing me, he could also have his eye on someone's children.

I would never forgive myself if a little girl disappeared, and I hadn't made a report. How easily someone could vanish and no one would know.

When we got home, I called the Ventura Highway Patrol and explained what had happened. They took the information and said thank you for the phone call.

A month later, I received a call from the officer that had taken the report. They had picked up the hairy bear on an "unrelated offense." The fact I had reported the incident was valuable to them for their case against him.

As I pedaled Oregon alone, you can understand my big sigh of relief every time a van pulled up and it was Gabriel in

our Love Machine. I can't let the memories of the scary
incident dwell in my mind. There will be many more lonely
roads in the days ahead.

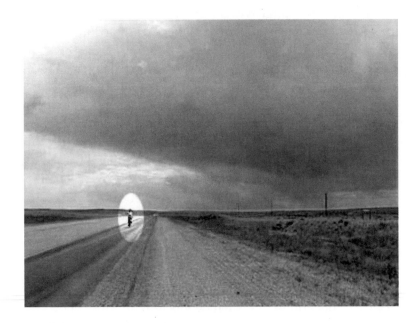

Day 7:
Baker City, OR to
Ontario, OR

83 miles

Hooray! What a fun day! I finally found something I was good at. I could coast!

After struggling up all those mountains in the freezing cold and then the blistering heat, I was now flying down the hills like everyone else. I had become accustomed to my niche as the "caboose" bringing up the rear. That day I had fun being one of the gang as we descended from the high desert.

The roads rolled downhill gradually. It wasn't a scary ride like snaking down a mountain with brakes on. Such a heavenly feeling – my bike was in "neutral" and all I had to do was steer.

Everyone was in a good mood. The past few days were ultimate survival ventures for me, and others had struggled too. Now we were enjoying our reward.

The weather was superb. Only the motion of my body generated the soft breeze on my face. Golden fields stretched forever. In the distance, I could see a huge blob of something. As I sailed down the hill and got closer, I realized it was a herd of cattle crossing the road. Several cowboys were waiting to stop us. They didn't want the cattle to be spooked. They asked us to get off our bicycles and follow them as they walked through the herd. There surely was a lot of "mooing" going on! There were hundreds of them, but they all behaved admirably.

The "easy" riding enabled my mind to mull over the interview I had in Baker last evening. The female reporter from the Baker City Herald was waiting at the first gas station as I rolled into town.

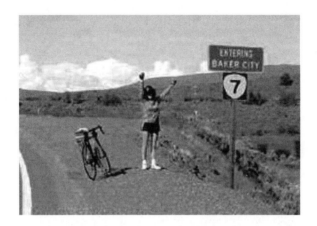

She asked questions and chatted with us for two hours. She was fascinated with the feat itself, and also with how I looked. What was age 67 supposed to look like? I guess not a woman in short shorts and Hanes Pantyhose trekking across America on a bicycle.

She wanted to know the details of our "route maps" and how we could find our way every day in uncharted territory. She looked at the sheet of paper and commented, "How can you make heads or tails out of this? Please help me understand."

I told her, "The most important item to look at is the mileage gauge. It said: 5.3 miles turn R on Main Street. Next item was .07 miles turn L into Holiday Inn. If you watch your odometer, you'd be prepared for a change or a new command. If not, you'd go sailing by and have to come back and look for the turn."

The reporter asked, "How do you keep track of so many things and still pay attention so you don't run into cars?"

"That's the catch," I said. "You have to be multi-tasking even on a bicycle. Some days we have as many as

twenty-five different commands to follow." I turned the sheet
over to show her the elevation graph on the back. "This shows
how many hills or mountains we have to climb. The elevations
or mountains on the graph are 'affectionately' called 'boobs.'
At a glance, you can see if it's a two or three 'boob' day or if
the riding would be relatively flat. Naturally, if it was a 'three
boob,' everyone would be groaning!"

After saying our goodbyes to the reporter, we looked
for our hotel. We almost missed dinner, because they were
having bicycle speed races on some of the downtown streets.
We wanted to stop and watch. I was hungry and hurting so
didn't stay too long. The ride plus a two-hour interview had
made for another long day!

I relished the present day's delicious rolling descent
into Ontario.

DAY 8:
ONTARIO, OR TO
BOISE, ID

62 MILES

What a way to start a day - riding through bucolic farming country on roads that seemed more like country lanes.

Peaceful is the perfect word to describe that extraordinary morning. On one side of the road was a corral with dozens of bison standing there acting like huge cattle. On the other side, a colt had so recently entered the world that its mother was still licking it and trying to help it get up on all four legs. Potatoes, onions and lettuce were growing in fields in the rolling hills.

Occasionally, I pedaled through small towns starting to wake up for the day. The next one caught my attention. It was "Star, Idaho." I pulled over, grabbed my phone and dialed.

I actually got Gabriel on the other end!

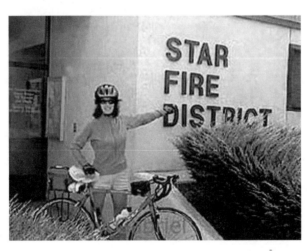

"I'm so excited—I'm in the town of Star. I'll wait here however long it takes for you to catch up. I didn't know there was a town by that name on the entire planet. My name was originally spelled with one 'r' and the second one was added when the family came to America. Also, my bicycle is named 'Starfire.' How perfect is that!"

The mileage for the day was only 62 miles so I could afford to hang around and wait. Gabriel wheeled the van in after an hour or so, grabbed his camera and off we went to investigate the town. We noticed the Star District Fire Station. When Gabriel and I stopped in to introduce ourselves, they were as amazed to meet a "Star" as I was to find their town.

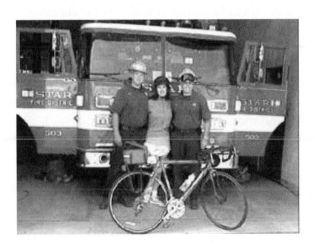

They couldn't believe I was pedaling across America and happily posed for pictures with me.

Kids gathered around to see what was going on. We were undoubtedly excitement for them in the little town. They had fun, too, clowning for the camera as Gabriel snapped photos.

After exploring the rest of Star, Gabriel filled me in on his morning. In the hotel elevator, he met a man who said to him, "You know, I was reading the Baker City Herald this morning over my cup of coffee. I read about this extraordinary 67 year-old woman who is pedaling her bicycle all the way across America. She must be something else – none of my friends could even pedal out of town and this town ain't very big."

Gabriel smiled, looked at the man and said, "Sir, the woman you were reading about is my wife!"

The man was astonished. He said, "Wait 'til I tell my friends I met the husband of this famous lady. You've really made my day."

They both had a good laugh over how they ended up in the same elevator.

I got all choked up as I realized I had pedaled across the entire state of Oregon and survived. Talk about a dream…

Entering Boise, we were routed through a residential area and past a luscious, green, rolling golf course. After the trials and tribulations of eight days on the road, I was ready for a day off; and thankful for the non-stressful day leading into civilization in the picturesque capitol city of Idaho.

Day 9:
Rest day in Boise, Idaho

Was I dreaming? We didn't have to hit the road at 6:15 am, rain or shine?

Our first rest day after pedaling eight days and traveling 613 miles was spent in Boise, the capitol of Idaho. As the day unfolded, it wasn't an idle day. It was a day to catch up on laundry, bicycle repairs and e-mails: things that can't be done on the road.

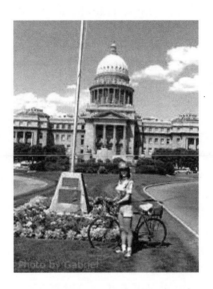

My first realization in the morning was how much my little toe hurt, the innocent toe I whacked on the nightstand shortly after we arrived here yesterday. It looked like a prism with all the colors of the rainbow showing up in various hues. Not pretty! The pain was excruciating. How was I ever going

49

to fit the fat toe into my shoe and make those pedals go around?

I asked the docs about it at breakfast. They assured me the only thing I could do was to tape it to the rest of my foot. The Technicolor toe had many miles to pedal and a !@#$%^#&%$*$@)* toe was not going to stop me!

How could I be so clumsy? I was going too fast, as usual, and didn't notice the nightstand protruding a few inches into the "walking area" in our motel room. My screams of pain probably resonated all over the city of Boise. I knew I was going to get teased that Gabriel was chasing me around the hotel room...she's finally off that bicycle for a day!

Now I'm trying to ride the impossible dream with a broken toe.

Even though it wasn't a day of road experiences, before the day was over, I found myself sitting in the governor's chair in his own private office!

When I left Santa Barbara, there wasn't time to get everything done. My pedals were for clip-on cleats, which terrify me. The clips on the bicycle shoes fit directly into holes in the pedals. When you twist your foot, you are completely locked onto the pedal until you untwist the foot to release the seal between shoe and pedal. I rode in my tennis shoes because of my fear of being locked onto my bicycle.

During the last multiple sclerosis charity ride in Santa Barbara, I had toe clips that also had straps on them to firmly hold my foot in place. One of the riders stopped immediately in front of me without warning as we came out of a rest stop onto a main highway. I braked to avoid landing on top of him; but there wasn't time to untangle my feet from the straps. I went over on my bike like the little old man in the yellow raincoat used to do on "Laugh-In."

That, however, was not funny. When I went over, my body went onto the road, and car tires roared by only a few feet from my head. I developed a real phobia about anything holding me tightly to my bicycle. My knees and legs were badly scraped and bleeding, but they healed. The fear caused by the car whizzing by my ear never did fade.

All the "real" cyclists have said I'll never finish the ride unless I use the conventional bicycle cleats that hold the foot tightly to the pedal. Supposedly, you gain thirty-five percent more power as your body and bike are locked together. Everyone has had spills while learning to unclip both feet before toppling over – especially difficult in an emergency stop. They still terrified me. It's one more part of me that will remain unconventional.

The day we left Santa Barbara, the media had a going-away luncheon for us. The Baron, who was the DJ on radio AM 1290 and in touch with me every day via his station, was instrumental in setting it up. There were hundreds of people, friends and media, to send us off in grand style. One gentleman came with a set of new red and black bicycle bags as a special gift to me.

My good friend, Susie, and her two sons were there. Several years ago she and her family invited me to go with them on my first charity ride, a 50-miler in the Solvang area. At the time, I had never thought cycling that many miles was possible. I hurt so badly when the day was over, it's a miracle I still owned a bicycle. It was the first building block; my friend didn't realize the seeds she had planted.

Susie brought me a baby blue long-sleeved bicycle shirt as a present and tucked in her bicycle shoes for extra "good luck." The shoes were half a size too big; but I put them in the van anyway as the "I'm with you" reminder they were meant to be.

I tried to slip my swollen toe into my own shoe, but there was no way it was going to fit. Susie's "too-big" shoes came to the rescue. Gabriel found them tucked in a corner in the van. My foot at least fit in the shoe. I hobbled over to the repair shop, replaced the clip-on pedals with a regular flat pedal and off I went, in pain, but back on my bike.

The unconventional combo of a "non-biker" pedal and the oversized bicycle shoes from a friend would get me over the next three thousand miles to Portsmouth, New Hampshire.

Gabriel was on his racy-looking bicycle. He had no intention of doing any long-distance riding but enjoyed the freedom of exploring the city with me on our bikes.

When we arrived in Boise yesterday, we were lost as usual. We knew our motel was not far from the landmark capitol building. We stopped a patrolman on the grounds of the capitol to ask for directions. He was kind enough to get us

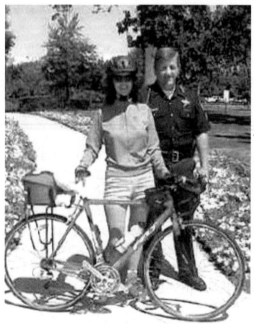

going in the right direction and took pictures with me. Then he said, "Come back tomorrow during normal working hours and go up to meet the governor."

We had never dreamed of doing anything like that. I
didn't think a governor would be accessible. But after all, the
nice policeman told us to do it. We parked our bicycles outside
and walked into the awesome marble building.

Everything else we'd seen since we started on the ride
across Oregon had been "country" but not that building. It was
elegant. We spoke with a guard at the door. I asked him to keep
an eye on our bicycles, confiding that I was cycling across
America.

He graciously explained how to find the governor's
office.

As we approached the secretary's office in the
governor's wing, we looked at each other. The shiny marble
floors, dark wooden doors and gold lettering with the state
seals were impressive.

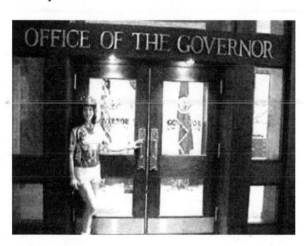

I whispered, "Should we be here?"

Gabriel said, "We're here. We might as well go in."

When we entered the office, a friendly secretary said,
"Hello. May I help you?"

Gabriel responded, "My sixty-seven year old wife is
pedaling her bicycle across America."

The secretary asked, "Did I hear you correctly? How can your wife be sixty-seven and look like she does? And, did I hear you say she was riding across America? I've never met anyone who has done anything so spectacular."

She continued, "The governor is out of the office for several days because of a herniated disc problem. I am sorry you will not be able to meet him. We have strict security rules about access to his office. But I'm so impressed with what you are doing, follow me."

She opened the door, led us up to his desk, pulled out his chair and motioned for me to sit down. She said, "Take as many pictures as you like. I'll take you sitting in the governor's chair with Gabriel standing beside you."

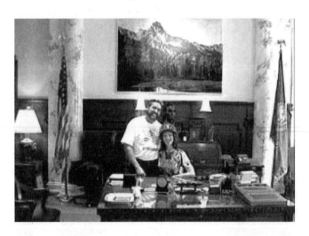

What an honor! What an experience! That was a completely unexpected thrill.

We floated out of the offices after extending many "thank yous" to the gracious secretary.

Everywhere I went, I felt admiration for what I was doing. That wasn't the intention of the ride, but it was gratifying to see and feel support for being a woman in good shape at the age of sixty-seven trying to accomplish a spectacular dream.

When we got back down to the main floor, the nice guard was still there. He said, "A severe storm is on the way and you are welcome to bring your bikes into the capitol building while it passes."

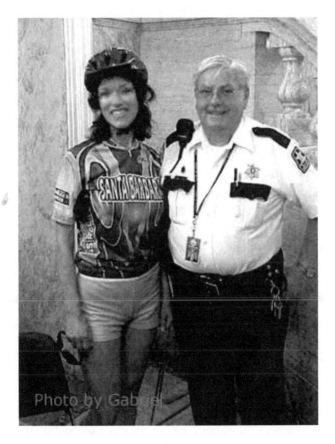

We were such naïve southern Californians. We thanked him and said, "We're not scared of a little rain." We should have listened and accepted his kind offer.

After we had pedaled about ten blocks, it started to sprinkle. No big deal. I had already been wet a few times on the ride. Then the sky opened up and it started "pouring

55

buckets" as we describe it in the Midwest. Lightning bolts streaked across the sky in every direction and thunder crashed down so close and loud that we were freaking out! We jumped off our bikes and waded to the curb. We tried to hide under the eaves of a building. The rain was blowing so intensely we were still getting soaked.

Gabriel dashed across the alley with his bicycle, but I was too slow and didn't make it. He was under the overhang next to a cement multi-story parking lot. I crawled into the raised brick flower box attached to the building and huddled there in the cramped space.

We watched the spectacular storm from those positions. The lightning, thunder, wind and rain lasted for an hour. It was awesome and scary. The streets flooded and water was running up and covering the sidewalks.

As the storm cell moved on, Gabriel ran out into the street to take some pictures. A big truck came by and made a "rooster fan" from the water, hitting him from the back while he was clicking away. It soaked him completely and the force of the water almost knocked his feet out from under him.

Now he knew about thunderstorms. Gabriel, being a native Santa Barbaran, had lived a sheltered life as far as the elements were concerned. We hopped back on our bicycles and leisurely pedaled back to our hotel.

At dinner that night the main topic was "Where were you when the big storm hit?" We cyclists had fanned out all over the city.

Can you believe on our day off we were still on our bicycles?

Day 10:
Boise, ID to
Mountain View, ID

51 miles

After our rest day in beautiful Boise, we had another treat, a short mileage day. It was a good day to stretch out and ride as fast as I could. I actually rode to the first sag stop, 23 miles, without stopping.

It was a long stretch, but I had a specific reason. We were riding on I-84, and the freeway had pros and cons. The good news was a nice, wide shoulder to ride on. The bad news was fast moving traffic, and the constant noise was frightening.

I tried to "hang behind" a friend who was willing to slow his pace so I could keep up. The biggest fear on the freeway was having a problem of any kind. If the sag was ahead (almost always for slow-poke me), it cannot turn around to come back. It has to find an exit, backtrack and catch up. Many extra miles would be added before help arrived.

It was a good thing my friend was my "friend." Guess who had a flat tire! I have only had two but my luck ran out. It was a rear tire again, and I still can't change it and get the gears on correctly. Dan pulled over with me into a burned out spot off the freeway. It looked like the best bet as there was heavy, dried grass all around which was usually full of stickers.

Dan put in my spare inner tube and the stem broke off as he inflated it. That was my only spare, so he put his on. He pumped it up and we shouted "Hooray."

Dan stepped back to admire his work and stepped on a "rolling rock" that tumbled him head over heels into the ditch. Rolling through the burned out area covered him with ashes from head to foot. He was a mess! We were hot and sweaty, so the ashes stuck like glue. I offered to wash his clothes when we got to our destination, but he declined. We were both giggling. He'd probably think twice before letting me tag after him again.

Chivalry still existed!

Because it was a short day, a repair clinic was slated in the afternoon. Appropriately for me, it was on "changing a tire." It's hard to believe it took an hour and a half to cover the subject, but it did.

We cyclists enjoyed some relaxation time around a gorgeous stone pool at the hotel.

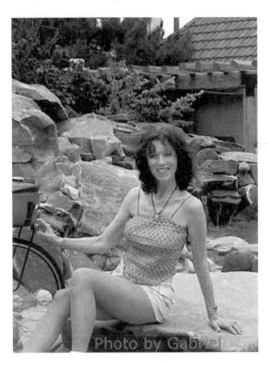

The first day on the road with my broken toe was a real bummer, but I did learn how to reposition my body on the bike to relieve some of the pressure. The pain was still incredible and it was impossible to walk on it.

A 97-mile day was next on the agenda, so I had to be in bed by 8:30 p.m. The early-to-bed hours were definitely a new experience.

Sounded like bedtime for a baby!

Day 11:
Mountain View, ID to
Twin Falls, ID
97 miles

       The day was almost another century, but the weather was so beautiful it made the riding easier. Gabriel and I met in Bliss – I didn't say we were in bliss even though we were – confusing? Bliss was a small town with two main attractions. I posed on and hugged them both; a bright red vintage fire truck, and a dinosaur whose head was at least twenty-five feet off the ground. We were in the Wild West! There were thousands of head of cattle keeping me company and talking to me. After some of the lonely roads, I was happy to be near anything that was alive!

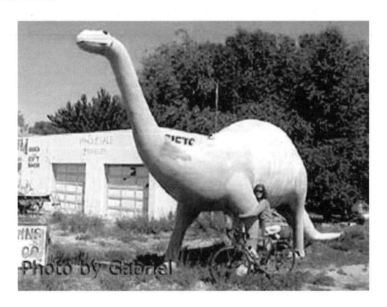

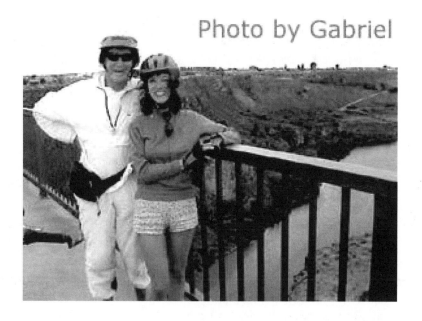

Photo by Gabriel

A huge suspension bridge soared out over Snake River Canyon below, as I got closer to Twin Falls. Looking down from the bridge, I saw a completely manicured golf course on the canyon floor. What a gorgeous sight from above. The wind played havoc with me again in the afternoon, but I knew I'd better get used to it.

Day 12:
Twin Falls, ID to
Burley, ID

38 miles

The short day was a gift. "Route rap" at 8:00 a.m.
meant no one left early. We were in Burley by noon (even me)!

Idaho was so mountainous; most of the residents lived
on the Snake River Plain. It extended almost from the
Oregon/Idaho border on the west to Yellowstone National Park
on the east. The lush, irrigated farmland stretched for miles
along the river. The frontage roads allowed us to ride leisurely
and enjoy the beauty and peace. We didn't have to cope with
noisy freeways or heavy traffic.

Because of the short travel day, Mike had a workshop
scheduled in the afternoon. It related to gears, drive-chains and
derailers, all the moving parts on the bicycles, and how to
properly care for them. Always something to learn!

There was a treat for me as we gathered for dinner—a
piano in the lobby. That was only the second one since we left
Santa Barbara. I played "Rhapsody in Blue" for everyone; and
even though my fingers were feeling stiff, the gang enjoyed it
immensely.

Our play-day culminated after dinner with a scavenger
hunt. My team didn't win, but we relaxed and had fun. What a
special group of people. We had been together almost two
weeks by now, and we felt like a big family.

Day 13:
Burley, ID to
Blackfoot, ID

110 miles

It's the old grade school story about the tortoise and the hare – I have gotten faster, but so has everyone else. They are still passing me by. There were four people who sagged at least part of the miles, but I pedaled every one!

It was going to be a l-o-n-g day. I was the second one out of the parking lot at 6:30 a.m. The first fifteen miles were easy, but then a horrible wind kicked up. By the time I got to the first sag stop about thirty miles down the road, my body was numb. The guys with big muscles were OK, but some of the others were struggling just as I was.

I called Gabriel, late in the morning, pleading, "Please, I need help and encouragement. The wind thrashed my body so thoroughly I don't have feelings in my limbs. I think I have 'hit the wall' as they say."

"Baby, hang in there. I'm many miles behind you as I stopped to buy fireworks for tomorrow night. I'm so excited to be able to do something for the gang. We can fire them here in Idaho, unlike California. You know what a big kid I am, and being able to do this makes me feel really good. I can't get to you for another hour so don't give up. I know this is a super long day. I love you and I'll be there with hot beans and weenies for you. I'll put them on the engine right now so they'll be warm."

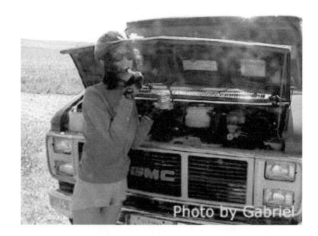

Photo by Gabriel

Idaho was definitely "meat and potatoes" with many cattle lots and huge barns to store potatoes. I've never seen so many potatoes. I'm used to buying them in a 10 pound plastic bag.

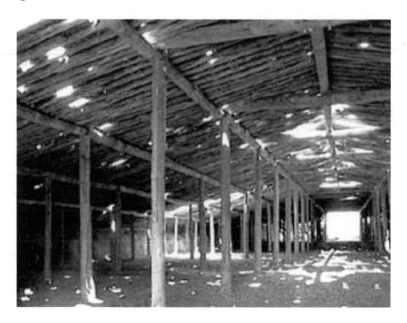

Along the way, we stopped to talk to an officer parked on the side of the road.

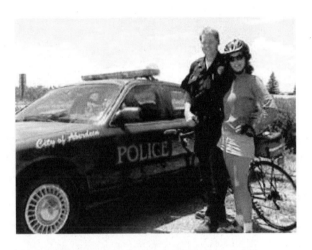

Gabriel asked," Can I take your picture with Patricia?"
He replied, "Sure."
I said, "It's OK to put your arm around me. One of my special Santa Barbara friends, Sergeant Dave Gonzales, is called the "The Singing Cop:"
The officer laughed. "That's what they call me! I just finished the lead roll of Captain VonTrapp in "The Sound of Music."
Never knew whom you'd meet out in the "boonies."

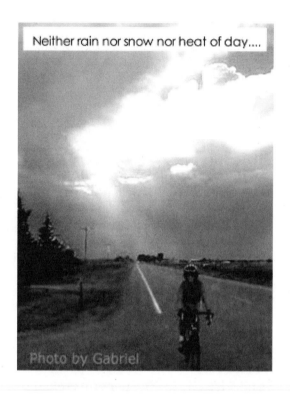

Neither rain nor snow nor heat of day....

Photo by Gabriel

In the late afternoon, a storm that had been threatening started to bear down on me. Thank goodness for Gabriel's hot lunch. I still had twenty miles to pedal, and it became a race to the finish. The lightning, thunder and black clouds chased me down the road. As I pedaled into Blackfoot and found our motel, the storm unleashed its fury. The motel was on the other side of a four-foot wall but the entrance was several hundred yards down the road. One of the cyclists already at the motel yelled at me, "Patricia, stop! I'm coming. I'll lift your bike over."

It started to pour as he picked up my bike and I scrambled my body over the wall. The wind was so strong we could hardly make it back to the motel.

The funny part (or not so funny) was that America By Bicycle had planned a treat for us, an outdoor barbecue on the motel patio. So much for that idea. They had to cram all of us into the hotel lobby in addition to the food tables. Sure brings back Nebraska memories of plans thwarted by Mother Nature. An hour later, the storm was gone, the sun came out, and peace in the heavens resumed.

Day 14:
Blackfoot, ID to
Idaho Falls, ID

34 miles

What fun! Not only was that one of the few short days, it was the 4th of July. We were usually intense from the moment we hit the road, but that day we didn't need to push. We spent the first hour decorating our bicycles. My red bike, shorts and turtleneck made it simple, as I was already half way there. Winding blue and white crepe paper around my spokes finished the patriotic look.

Gabriel was so excited as no one knew he had hundreds of fireworks in the van from yesterday's shopping spree. He was ready for a spectacular evening.

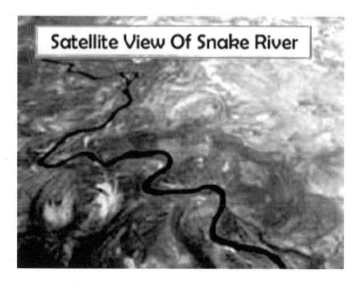

Satellite View Of Snake River

We all savored the easy day, knowing what was in store for us the next two days, Teton Pass and Togwotee Pass. Was I capable? None of us could comprehend or predict what that incredible challenge actually would feel like.

Rolling into Idaho Falls was a feast for the eyes and ears. The Snake River had been dammed up to make spectacular short waterfalls as you entered over the bridge into the city. The sounds of rushing water were everywhere and the parkways along the river were luscious shades of green.

When Gabriel pulled up in the van, he had no idea his plans for a great evening had been sabotaged. Idaho Falls had a city council composed of Mormons, and they had banned all fireworks for the 4th of July because it was a Sunday. Gabriel was never disrespectful toward anyone's religious beliefs, but he surely didn't agree with that ruling!

It was his chance to be a big kid and do something spectacular for all the "fireworks-lovers." He shook his head in disbelief that he had a van full of happiness for many people and had been gunned down by a council in a state where the fireworks *were* legal, unlike California.

Obviously, he couldn't return fireworks and get his money back. No one had bothered to tell him about the Mormon ruling when he purchased them. He knew he couldn't fight "city hall," and also couldn't "sneak" them off as our leaders would have shut him down. When we rolled into a town, we all had to be exemplary citizens—even if it squelched our fun.

Gabriel's disappointment was assuaged a bit by an interview with an exceptionally nice reporter from KDIK Newswatch 3. We chatted and took pictures for two hours and had such a good feeling about Idaho Falls in spite of the fireworks debacle.

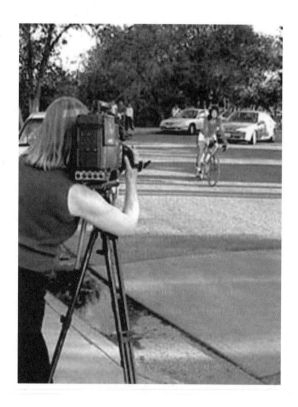

What a bummer his celebration idea had turned out to be! He also had to find a way to dispose of them. When we returned to our third floor room after dinner, he saw an apartment complex from our window and noticed some older kids playing around. He went down to find them.

"Hi there—how you doin? Would you kids like some free fireworks?"

"Are you jiving us? What's the catch?"

"No catch. I found out I can't shoot these off tonight because it's Sunday, and I don't want to be driving around tomorrow with them in my van."

"Sure, we'll take them. We can set some off tonight before we get caught and then have lots of fun tomorrow. Gee, thanks."

They thought it was Christmas in July.

When Gabriel got back to our room, he said, "Look out the window. You're going to see a few fireworks. At least I made some kids happy."

Knowing what was on the agenda tomorrow; I was almost asleep but did see a few shooting stars out of my half-closed eyelids. Happy 4th of July!

Day 15:
Idaho Falls, ID to
Jackson, WY

88 miles

I woke feeling apprehensive. I knew it would be a day of torturous physical challenges as we started our ascent over the Continental Divide. It would take two days: Teton Pass the first day and Togwotee Pass the second. Could I handle it? It was uncharted territory for most of us. Riding a bicycle over the Rocky Mountains sounded like a fairy tale.

Everyone had been talking about it for days. It was interesting how the leaders of the group referred to the day, but didn't say anything about it except the last three miles were "extremely steep." It was like having your first root canal; nobody told you what it was *really* like. It was something you *had* to do.

The altitude was a concern for many of the cyclists. There was nothing you could do to prepare for it. Stories were circulating.

Janet volunteered, "One of my best friends, an excellent climber, had to be carried off the mountain last week because of the altitude. He was an athlete in top condition but had trouble breathing. He felt so helpless."

Nathan spoke up, "I read as much as I could before I started the ride. You better get off the mountain quickly if you feel dizzy, nauseous, or disoriented. There is nothing else you can do except get back to a lower elevation so your body gets the oxygen it needs."

Carol added, "If I start getting woozy, I hope there's a sag around to get me out of there pronto. I don't want to ruin the entire day feeling sick."

We would have to climb almost 10,000 feet to get over the Continental Divide. How was *my* body going to react? I did not have a clue. Imagine dealing with the above symptoms and being on a bicycle. The sag was the only option for those overcome by altitude sickness.

I hoped my angel would take care of me so that I wouldn't end up in the sag.

I was on the road at 6:15 a.m. to be in the front pack of riders. I knew from experience they would pull away from me in a few miles, but I had a head start on the day. At least I thought I did.

It didn't take long to get out of the town. As the last stoplight turned green and I pushed hard on my left pedal, my foot kept going and slammed into the ground. I yelled, "I need help! Something happened to my pedal."

Terry and Joe pulled up and stopped.

Terry inquired, "Patricia, what are you doing to yourself. Isn't one broken toe enough?"

Joe piped up. "Come on Terry. Didn't you hear she broke her toe because her husband was chasing her around the hotel room? That sounded more exciting than slamming your foot into the ground at a stoplight."

I said, "Come on you guys, please. Tell me what's wrong."

Terry examined the pedal. "Sorry, Patricia. I can't fix it. The toe clip broke off at the joint. You're going to need the mechanic and the sag to get you going again. We're facing tremendous climbs today, and you won't be able to climb without a new clip. You can creep along until the sag catches up to you. Sorry I had to deliver the bad news."

"Thanks, guys. At least I know what's wrong, and I didn't break another toe."

73

Several riders stopped to see what was happening. They delivered the same diagnosis.

My only choice was to ride slowly without pressure on the pedal so my foot would not thrust forward. I didn't need a broken or sprained ankle. My broken little toe was a real bummer; it hurt all the time. How could I have been so clumsy!

I called the sag, told them where I was and that I would be continuing at a snail's pace. When they caught up, we found a place where we could both pull over.

The van had a supply of almost everything so the part was available, but it took the mechanic half an hour adapting it to fit my particular pedal.

I was pacing back and forth on the shoulder of the road, happy the mechanic was there but wishing he would hurry up.

I was already forty-five minutes behind everyone else, and the day was only starting. I had lost fifteen minutes riding slowly and another thirty minutes for the repair. I didn't need a set back on one of the most difficult days on our itinerary.

By now, everyone had passed me except Bill who rides the two-wheeler recumbent bicycle. He had a hard time pedaling up the hills; he was normally in the back with me, the diesel. We're the backend buddies out on the road.

When he came up behind me, he yelled, "Patricia, I'm so sorry, but I have to pass you and keep going! I don't know how I'm going to be able to make the long day and the terrific climb at the end."

I yelled back, "I know Bill, I understand. I'll be OK." What I was really thinking was *Oh @#$%^#&% -- there goes my lifeline*! No matter how many hours I had ridden alone, it was a comfort to know Bill was usually back there "somewhere."

74

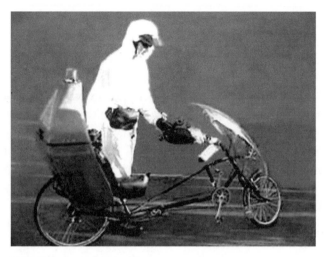

Now there was no one.

Finally, the mechanic said, "OK Patricia. You're ready for the road. Don't get a speeding ticket."

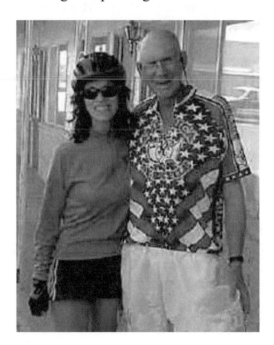

"Me? That's really funny! I'm glad you were available and could fix the problem. I know you worked as fast as you could. Thanks again."

It didn't take long to get out of civilization and into the most barren, desolate country one could imagine. I grew up in Nebraska in a cornfield where everything was green and lush in the summer. With no vegetation, I felt more vulnerable and alone when there was nothing alive but me. I would have to endure many more miles of bleakness as we crossed Wyoming and South Dakota.

The day was significant in another way. My friend, Jorge, a fine musician I had known and played with for years, had made a special tribute on a power-point show concerning my adventure across America, the reason for the ride and the music scholarship at Santa Barbara City College. He used a gorgeous shot of the Grand Teton Mountains on the cover page. I had never been to the Tetons before, but had heard about their magnificent beauty.

Somehow, the incident was permanently etched in my mind. I never dreamed the picture would be instrumental in keeping my sanity.

Pedaling in the vacuum of the desert seemed like an eternity. If you are in a car, the hundred miles of nothing would pass in less than an hour and a half, but on a bicycle, it was the entire day! Don't even ask what you needed to do when you had to go to the bathroom. There was no corner service station available.

I was riding into a terrific headwind, so no matter how hard I tried to push ahead, the wind kept holding me back.

The only other person in the entire landscape was Bill, who was way ahead by now. Occasionally, I could see Bill, a tiny speck in the far distance. I had no hope of closing the gap between us. His tiny speck of life kept getting smaller.

76

As another storm approached and surrounded me, I frantically tried to call Gabriel, but phone reception was zero. With such a sparse population, technology wasn't a part of the landscape.

A book I had scanned before I left on the ride dealt with the mental aspect of handling such an adventure. I remembered reading that mental stress caused more bicyclists to give up than fatigue, saddle sores or aching muscles.

I frantically raced along, my mind focusing on the mountains in the distance. Those were the mountains I had fallen in love with via Jorge's photograph. I concentrated on riding into the stunning picture that was so vivid in my mind. My terror and panic were intense. *THERE WAS NOBODY THERE BUT ME…at least that's what I thought.*

We often say, "I'm alone in my car" or "home alone." That in no way described what it felt like being alone in the desert. When I was in the depths of utter despair, a magnificent moment was about to happen.

An angel appeared out of the heavens. It was so dramatic against the blackness of the storm clouds. It was Jorge's angel, my friend who had given me the photograph.

The wind, the lightning and thunder, and the blackened sky were still the same. When the angel's wings enfolded my body, they protected me from the fear of reacting to the impending storm and my complete isolation.

Gabriel finally came along in our van and found me riding down the lonely road. He had no idea I had encountered mechanical problems that put me behind everyone else. He was earlier than usual; it was only a little after eleven o'clock.

He had seen the ominous storm clouds and felt he should start out sooner. He had loaded up quickly. He recalled our heavy van being pushed around on the road by the extreme 50-mph swirling winds. He was worried about me.

When I told him about the angel wings protecting me, I'm sure he thought I had gone over the edge. I had never had an angel experience like that.

It wasn't that I didn't believe in angels. As a musician, I had played and sung in churches of almost every denomination. I felt I was a religious person, but real angel experiences had seemed a little "far out" to me.

My friend Jorge had endured much pain because of severe back problems. Dealing with it constantly had made him strong. Somehow, his strength was transferred to me through his angel so I could continue. It was amazing how it all tied into a photograph of the Tetons, where we were at the moment.

Shortly after Gabriel arrived, the huge threatening clouds started to blow off. We saw some frightening bolts of lightning and heard the thunder crash. The rain never came though so I didn't even get wet.

The climbing started in the early afternoon. So much had already happened; I almost forgot that this would be one of the toughest days of the entire ride. Now, however, Gabriel was somewhere near in the "Love Machine."

As we hit the last three miles, I understood why no one talked about the climb. Half of the group would have given up before they started the day.

Even the Love Machine was chugging and working hard.

Gabriel drove ahead of me and around the next corner, out of sight, to give me a target as the road snaked up the mountain. I stopped many times in between. I had no granny or spinning gear on my bike – the extra low gear that lets your legs go around easily even though you travel only a short distance. When it was so steep that I couldn't physically turn the pedals anymore, I hopped off my bike, let my legs refuel for a minute, got back on and rode up another few feet or yards. It was incredibly grueling, but I would not give up.

I never have dwelled on the number of years I have been on the earth; but it did cross my mind that 67 years may have been a handicap under such a stressful and demanding situation. There were a few other cyclists in my age bracket; but I was the real greenhorn. One of the older men had ridden over 10,000 miles in the six months before the ride started. I never even got close to the first thousand.

Many of the group walked their bikes part way up the climb. Some didn't even attempt it and pushed their bikes up the entire three miles. Others were suffering high altitude symptoms and hitched rides in the two sag wagons.

I refused to walk an inch. No matter how slow I was, I pedaled all the way to the top. I had a dream! Luckily, my body didn't scream about the lack of oxygen. I huffed and puffed as I normally would.

What an incredible feeling when I spotted my favorite sign close to the top, a truck tipped sideways and downhill percentage written on it. I knew I was going to succeed. After a little more pedaling, I hopped off my bike and gave the sign a big hug. Gabriel got the next hug. He was already at the top with the Love Machine.

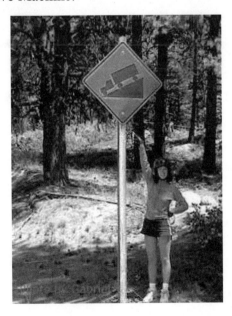

I had conquered one of the two tremendous climbs to get over the Rocky Mountains. What a feeling of sheer power to know I had done something so seemingly impossible.

I knew many were watching me, including my fellow cyclists, the media and friends. Teton Pass was definitely a "biggie." Was the 67-year-old "bicycle broad" in the Hanes hosiery and short shorts with her "boy" going to have the stuff it takes to conquer a mountain such as that?

They all found out.

There was an incredible downhill prize awaiting me. Whee!

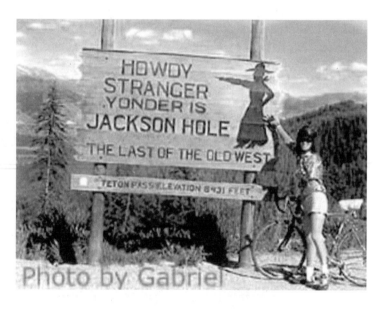

DAY 16:
JACKSON, WY TO
DUBOIS, WY

88 MILES

BEAR LUNCHES ON BICYLIST – could that be me? I liked being in the headlines, but I wasn't interested in being the entrée. Now I had something else to worry about besides pedaling up all those mountains.

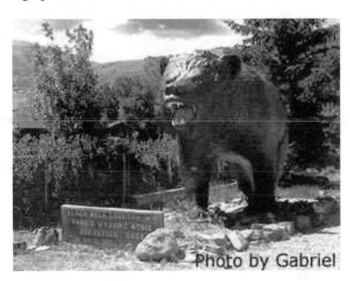

Photo by Gabriel

When I stopped at a small lodge around noon, I saw a huge flat bed truck in the parking lot. I thought there was a big metal barbecue tied on the truck bed. I noticed some guys standing around chatting, so I went over to be friendly. As I got closer, I smelled a horrible stench coming from the area.

81

I said, "Hello. That metal container is the biggest barbecue I've ever seen."

"Ma'am, that's not a barbecue. That's a bear trap."

"You're teasing me, I hope."

"No, Ma'am, I'm not teasing. We got a call from the lodge this morning saying there was a bear in the vicinity; and it had been sighted several times close to the road."

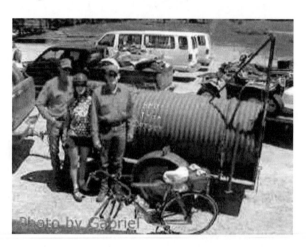

Photo by Gabriel

Gulp! You can imagine how that made me feel. I still had memories of my stalker, "hairy bear," in his rusty van with the bullet holes and my fear of being snatched by him.

Now, I had to worry about being snatched by a real bear.

I asked, "Do they really attack people? I'm riding my bicycle across America and I'm usually riding alone. Are they aggressive?"

"Ma'am, we can't answer that question. Bears are unpredictable. When we get a call, we try to trap them. We bait them with decomposing venison, and the bears really go for it."

"Is that the awful smell?"

"Yep, the venison is in the pickup over there. Then we take them to a higher elevation where there are less people and let them out. We're not here to harm them."

"Oh great. That's exactly where I'm going when I take off on my bicycle, *up* the mountain. I hope I don't have enough meat on me to be enticing."

The story of the bear sighting circulated among the cyclists. When I got to the sag stop, two cyclists were still there.

John said, "Patricia, the bear was looking for you, but he got tired of waiting; so he left. He heard rumors that you're usually the last one to check in."

"Thanks, John. Your comment isn't even funny. Would you like to be in my shoes for a day, a woman out here alone? You probably don't even know what fear feels like."

"No, I can't even imagine the feeling," John said. "Patricia, we all give you credit for having the guts to do something like this and for hanging in there every day until you get to the destination. There is a lot of admiration for what you are accomplishing."

"Thanks, John. Those words mean a lot to me. I *am* going to get to the east coast. If I meet the bear, I'll tell him to get out of my way."

Teton Pass had been conquered. Togwotee was a different climb. The ascent was an extremely steep forty-five mile incline. That's a lot of pedal pushing.

I've mentioned eternity climbs before, but Togwotee was the granddaddy of them all. Gabriel was staying closer, as I struggled up the mega mountain.

Talk about determination. It was an incredibly long afternoon of push, pedal and rest for a minute, again and again.

The closer I got to the top, the more I was tantalized by the reward – flying down the other side. I had to keep my mind in gear too!

I kept feeding my will to succeed by looking behind me each time I slipped off my bike to rest for a minute. I truly felt like the "Queen of the Hill" as the vistas rolled away as far as I could see.

Every day had been a struggle, some more than others. As I looked at the entire picture of riding America, crossing the Rocky Mountains at almost 10,000 feet was definitely the pinnacle of the trip.

When I started on the last ten miles, Gabriel started driving up to the top occasionally, coming back down and telling me, "Baby, the road looks exactly like the one you're on. You've pedaled this far. You can make it the rest of the way."

He played teaser games with me – only five more miles – four more…

Every time Gabriel came back down to me, he opened the cooler and made sure I ate something. That was not the time for me to be out of fuel.

As I approached the last mile, my mind tumbled over so many thoughts. How could I possibly conquer such a mountain? I knew there were cars that never made it over the passes.

Gabriel was getting so excited. He knew how close I was. He could hardly wait to dial back to Santa Barbara with the news "Patricia pedaled over the Continental Divide at 9,683 feet. She may be tired, but she's still alive!"

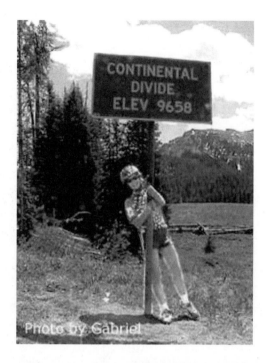

As I spotted my favorite sign with the leaning truck, I wondered if I could coast to the Atlantic. After I pushed those last few pedals that took me to the top, I ran over and gave the Togwotee Pass sign a big hug. About twenty feet away was the sign "Continental Divide." I had studied about the Rocky Mountains in my old Nebraska schoolhouse; but didn't realize until that moment that the two signs were almost side-by-side.

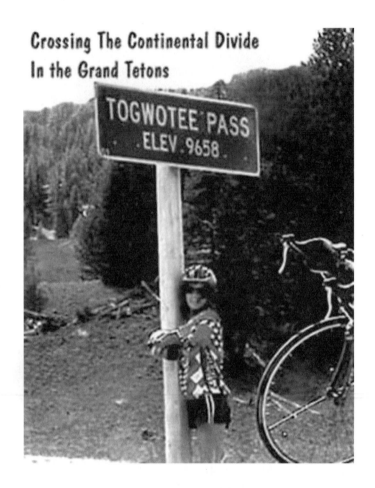

Crossing The Continental Divide
In the Grand Tetons

TOGWOTEE PASS
ELEV. 9658

Gabriel took pictures to commemorate the enormous accomplishment. Then we noticed some leftover snow under the trees. We finished our celebration with a snowball fight.

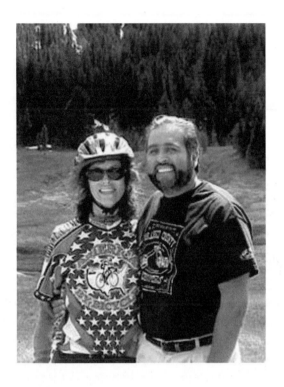

What else could you expect from two Californians?

Day 17:
Dubois, WY to
Riverton, WY

79 miles

After surviving the last two days, I didn't know what was coming next. The route map mileage was a sizable day in anyone's language. Seemed to me as though we should have deserved a rest! The good news was the notation that we would drop 800 feet in altitude in the first 30 miles on the road.

Being in "cruise control" for a few hours was the perfect time to reflect on the events of the last two days. The exhilaration of knowing I had pedaled over the Rocky Mountains and had survived was awesome. I almost felt giddy. It has burned a memory on my mind and soul to know anything is possible if I concentrate on hanging in there – no matter what the odds. Being successful those last two days was extremely powerful. Not many people can say they have ridden a bicycle over the Continental Divide at almost 10,000 feet. We didn't coast to the Atlantic from there, but I knew I could and would face whatever challenges came along.

As we dropped in altitude, the topography changed dramatically to red rocks and sagebrush. The road extended far beyond what the eye could see—the usual picture in most minds of what Wyoming looks like.

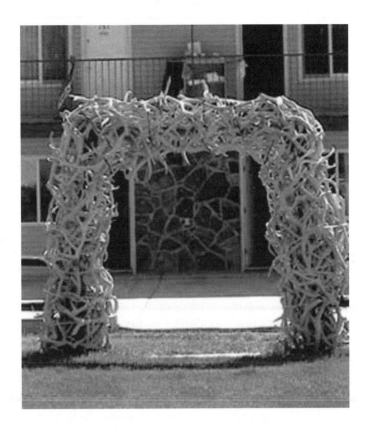

    As I rolled into Riverton, there was no doubt it was
cowboy country, with arches made entirely of antlers! The Big
Wind and Little Wind rivers converged there, much as the
history of the Old West and the New West have melded into a
town full of character in the hub of Wyoming.

Day 18:
Riverton, WY to
Casper, WY

120 miles

"Small town, America" has now taken on a new meaning. If there was a debate over where it was, I think I found the winner.

I struggled all morning against the wind, I was a twig being whipped every which way and constantly fighting to keep my bicycle upright. My body needed a break.

I approached a wide spot in the road and found a welcoming sign that said Hiland, "Population 10." That was stretching it. We found out the actual number of residents was two. That surely had to be the smallest town anywhere. Before the day was over, it was possibly a town of only "one."

We'll never know.

One hundred twenty miles was the longest day on our agenda so far. How did I cope mentally? I played tricks on my brain to keep from being overwhelmed. The extreme winds and heat added to the physical load of the day. I divided the miles into "bars" of ten miles each. As I pedaled along, I concentrated only on the number of bars. I needed twelve. That sounded better than 120 miles!

Bicycling the first thirty miles into a horrible headwind almost wiped me out in the first couple of "bars." I didn't think I was going to get to count to 12. The wind felt like a big hand pushing on my face and body that would not let go. One of the larger male cyclists told me to get directly behind him to break the force on me. He slowed his pace down, so I could keep up with him and draft behind him. Without him, I don't think I would have made it.

After the sag stop, the wind abated for a bit as it changed direction. My friend went on his way. Ominous black clouds were brewing in the distance. They started to get closer. I frantically dialed Gabriel; and thank you, angel, I got a connection. When I told him where I was and that a storm was threatening, he quickly packed up and got on his way.

It was the mileage problem again. On such a long day, I always had to worry about getting picked up by the sag wagon. They needed to keep their chicks a little closer together in case of an emergency. One hundred twenty miles was a lot of distance for two vans to cover. If they knew Gabriel was in touch with me, they would leave me alone.

Gabriel had come up behind me several miles back. I was looking for a spot to take a break, so we pulled over together. My map noted a tiny town a few miles ahead, so Gabriel took off. When I got there, he had cold water for me and pulled snacks out of the cooler. Because of the long, windy day, I had to "eat and run." As I put my gloves on, Gabriel said, "Go on ahead. I want to take a look inside the little store. I'll be right behind you."

I hadn't gone in the store, but I could see it was tiny. Forty-five minutes passed without Gabriel coming up beside me. How long could it possibly take to shop and look around? If he bought everything in the store, it could be rung up in half an hour.

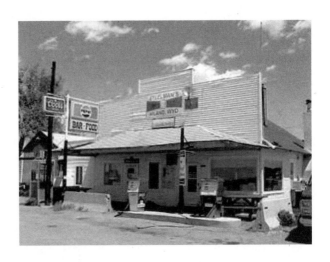

Where was he?

The long, lonely road stretched out forever and there was nobody on it. A helicopter that appeared in the distance was coming my direction. That was really strange. *What would he be doing out here in this nothing?* Then I heard sirens and an ambulance coming towards me on the highway. *Could they be looking for my hubby?* My heart and stomach were getting a panicky feeling. I had no idea what was going on and no phone service to find out.

Here I was again, all alone in the middle of nowhere and feeling helpless. Gabriel should have caught up to me an hour ago. There was nothing I could do but keep riding forward. I couldn't turn around and go back to look for him, I had 120 miles to pedal. Did he have an accident? With whom? There weren't even any other cars around.

I was really getting scared. I stopped for a drink and looked behind me. The road stretched forever and it was empty.

I rode another half hour, getting more and more frantic. The ambulance sailed by me. The helicopter zipped over my head.

92

My heart was beating erratically. Was my husband in the ambulance? Was he in the helicopter?

I pulled over off the highway and sat there on my bike with tears streaming down my face. Any energy left after fighting the wind and heat drained out of my body.

There can't be any feeling that was "more alone."

Oh my God. What now? I stroked the golden angel pinned on my turtleneck. Gabriel had given it to me shortly after we started dating. I never went anywhere without it. There had been many times when it was a comfort to me out there in the land of nowhere.

Why was Gabriel letting me be out here alone? He, and only he, knew how scared and lonely I got in the desert. I tried to portray self-assurance, because I wanted to finish my dream, but where in the hell was he?

He had better have a good excuse!

Between sobs and feeling sorry for myself, I heard a faint rumble and purr coming up behind me. A car! Not only was it another human being, it was Gabriel in the beautiful blue Love Machine. My heart was racing!

He pulled over and jumped out of the van. "Baby, I'm so sorry to leave you stranded here alone – again – and making you worry about me."

He continued, "You'll never believe this one. Half of the little town back there had a heart attack. It was happening while I was in the store trying to find more beans and weenies to heat up for your lunch. I didn't even know what was going on at first. Before you pedaled in, I had talked to some of the cyclists who were ready to take off again. They had tried to get food at the store's tiny kitchen. The problem was the owners got overwhelmed by so many people coming in at once. They were used to only a carload or a trucker or two."

93

With so few stops along the route, 45 cyclists had hit the store within a few hours and the owners couldn't cope. The cyclists were in a hurry because of the long day. They couldn't be patient. Many of them grumbled and went on without food. With 120 miles on the agenda, you have to keep pushing, even if you are an experienced cyclist.

"When I entered the store," Gabriel continued, "there was a lady behind the counter. I thought she was acting weird, but then I thought W*ho wouldn't in this God-forsaken place.* She was obviously stressed and anxious, but she was still trying to take care of business and help me. When I first noticed her nervousness and anxiety, I thought maybe she was afraid of me. Being a dark skinned Hispanic, I felt I stood out in white Middle America. In between times she would disappear into the back of the store. When she reappeared, she'd look out the window and scan the sky. That happened a few times. I finally asked her if she was OK."

She replied, "I'm looking for the helicopter. My husband is having a heart attack. If they don't get here quickly, he'll probably die."

Gabriel said it was the most unbelievable scene. She was trying to hold her composure and take care of business even though she was extremely worried about her husband. I suppose in that hostile environment, every customer was important. She must have been so trained to take care, even during a catastrophe, that the show went on.

Gabriel knew he couldn't leave. He said, "Go back to your husband. I'll watch for the helicopter."

When it approached, Gabriel guided it down. The pilot jumped out and shouted above the din of the whirling blades, "Stay where you are and make sure no one comes close to the rotors. I need to leave it running to enable a quick departure."

94

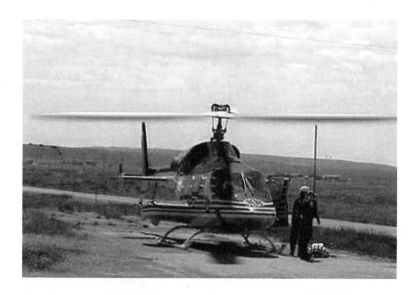

The paramedics were trying to stabilize the victim but he needed hospitalization – fast. After only a few minutes, the pilot and the medics appeared with the stricken man on a stretcher, loaded him on the helicopter and took off.

Gabriel looked at his watch. He was in the midst of so much drama; he could hardly believe an hour and a half had passed. He realized I was probably frantic, because I couldn't possibly know what was happening.

If I had left him at a shopping mall, many hours could have elapsed, as he loves to shop. At the tiny store, the time lapse made no sense.

I was sorry for the heart attack victim but so relieved that Gabriel was okay.

We still had many miles to go. The next stop was Hell's Half Acre. What a bizarre site in the barren land. It looked like a mini-version of the Grand Canyon with vivid colored rocks and jagged depths. It was obviously a tourist attraction with a funky, western café perched on the rim of the canyon.

Each day was a new adventure and that one included a
surprise for me – a gorgeous old upright piano in the café.
    I couldn't wait to get my fingers on the keys. Not only
was I lonesome for a piano, I wanted to see if my hands still
worked. The left one in particular was victim to "biker's hand."
The muscles had been contracted for so many hours, day after
day; they wouldn't release and allow the fingers to straighten
out completely. My hands worked but not well. I was so happy
to be making music that I didn't care.

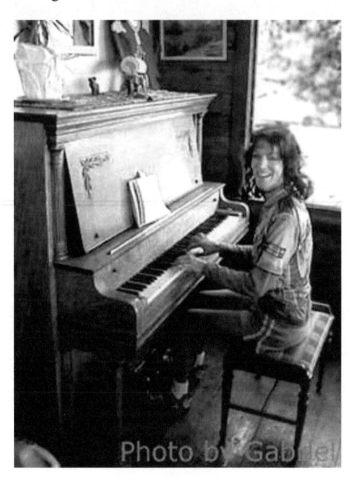

After a delicious lunch there, Gabriel and I stepped outside again and were almost blown away. The erratic wind never stopped. I never knew from which direction the next gust of wind would be coming.

When I got into the twelfth bar of my newly devised mile-counting system, I was exhilarated to know I was approaching Casper. I pedaled into town with my hands still gripping as hard as I could. A stoplight cost me any forward momentum to counteract the gusts of wind. My bike and I suddenly blew over into the gutter. Thank God I didn't have clip-ons. I was able to jump off quickly, or my ankle would have been crushed between the bike and the cement curb. I continued a few more yards down the road, and the same thing happened again. Unbelievable!

Ahead was a big, long bridge that spanned all the railroad tracks below. Gabriel had driven across with the traffic flow while I was picking myself up out of the gutter – twice. As I rode across the bridge, another huge gust blew me over again. This time it pinned my bicycle and me up against the bridge railing. The railing wasn't very tall, and it was frightening to look down at all the trains below. I couldn't move until the gust let up. Gabriel had already parked at the other end and saw what was happening to me. He could only wait as I peeled myself off the railing and started pedaling again.

We finally found our way to the motel. Everyone had finished eating by the time we got to the restaurant. We ordered our dinner and as the cyclists left, the fact we had all ridden 120 miles wasn't even mentioned. All the talk was about the wind! Even the best cyclists were saying, "What a day."

I smiled. I had pedaled it too!

Day 19:
Rest day in Casper, WY

I thought I was hallucinating. Nine days of pedaling without a break was too much. When I awoke and looked out our window, I saw the most amazing sight - palm trees, ferns, waterfalls, begonias, impatiens, and lilies... We were in a Holiday Inn completely enclosed under a huge dome like a snow globe. The restaurants, pools, rooms, and recreation areas were all covered. The result was a tropical paradise.

I forgot we were staying in a Holidome, something we Californians knew nothing about. That was how the rest of America survived when the weather was cruel (quite often in those parts). It looked like home, including the same kinds of flowers and fauna growing in our Santa Barbara gardens. As I blinked my eyes, I did remember rolling in here late last night after fighting the wind for 120 miles. There wasn't much left of me.

During the last nine days we had experienced the highest and longest challenges of the entire journey. If you threw in the constant wind and erratic gusts for a little spice, you got the picture.

Normal chores such as laundry and e-mail took up most of the day. We absorbed the atmosphere by leaving our motel room door open. Our room was on the ground floor, so the gardens were directly outside the door. It was a rest day for the body, soul and senses.

While strolling through the gardens, we met a nice family and their kids who were in the area for All-Star soccer tournaments. The family lived in another part of Wyoming. When I commented about the struggles of riding in the wind day after day, the father said, "We like the wind. People come here to visit and see how much property they can buy for their dollars, so they move here. Then when they **find out** what the wind and the weather are really like, they move **away**. There are less than 450,000 people in the entire state **and** we like it that way. Let the wind blow!"

    To each his own!

Day 20:
Casper, WY to Lusk, WY
106 miles

Here is Gabriel's description of the day as he wrote it for the website:

"Today was hell. 106 miles of nothing as far as the eye could see. I caught up with Patricia about 11:30. She was frantic, hot, tired and lonely as everyone else was far gone. She had tears in her eyes, as the heat and headwind were just about unbearable."

Amen! I thought. A perfect slant on the day. The only observation added was that the ups and downs of the road weren't apparent when driving a car in the desert. I felt every one of them on a bicycle. When the wind was not ferocious, there was a tiny bit of rest time when I could coast. With the terrific wind, it was necessary to pedal even going down hill. I fought for every pedal the entire day. Somehow, I made it.

I still have my dream!

Day 21:
Lusk, WY to
Hot Springs, SD

92 miles

"How can you leave me here in this heat? I have twenty miles to climb to the top, and I'm so hot I think I'm going to explode. I need help. Please spray me with water. I've been waiting for you to come along for hours. Don't leave me out here alone."

I had pulled off the road as I couldn't go an inch further. It was already over a hundred degrees at midday. Of course, I had hot tears running down my cheeks. There was no other way to vent my frustration.

Gabriel leaned out of the window of the Love Machine. "Baby, I don't know what I'm going to do. I have this man with me who needs to get up over the mountain to get a tire for his camper. His wife and two kids are about forty miles back and burning up from the heat. What do you expect me to do?"

I sobbed, "You're going to have to decide. I'm going to die out here if you don't keep my clothes soaked. I can't go any further without you."

The temperature had already been in the 80's at six in the morning when I started out. It had not cooled down during the night as it usually did. I knew I was going to be in trouble. The good news: the highway was in fantastic shape without a pothole in sight. The bad news: The people responsible for placing the "rumble bumps" – the washboards built into the cement to alert drifting drivers – must never have been on a bicycle. Instead of being placed on the edge of the auto lane,

101

they were in the shoulder on the two-foot strip we had to ride on. Each one was eight feet long, and they were placed about twenty feet apart. There was no place for the bicyclist except on the highway or off the road in the dirt. Riding a bicycle on a rumble bump made it shake so violently you couldn't control the steering.

As I crossed over another state line, I yelled, "Hello, South Dakota, you're my fourth state to bicycle across." There was no one around to hear me, but it felt good.

Aside from the heat, I was cruising along, as the highway was desolate and smooth riding. Gabriel was not around, yet, so I stopped at a tiny shopping center where the sag stop was set up and chatted with other cyclists about the challenge ahead of us.

Where was my honey? I had specifically asked him to be there, as we had been warned about climbing the mountain in the extreme heat. I had to move on. There was no other way to get to Hot Springs. Actually, the town was named for the mineral springs surrounding it, not the degrees on the thermometer. Made me wonder!

Gabriel had quite an experience being a Good Samaritan that morning before he caught up to me. He saw a camper parked on the shoulder with a man standing alongside. As he had done many times traveling across America, he pulled over.

"Hi there. My name is Gabriel. Looks like you've got a problem."

"Thanks so much for stopping. My name is John. I have a flat. The camper is so low, my jack won't fit underneath to raise it so I can change the tire. I tried to call AAA, but there's no phone service out here. I'm desperate and afraid for my family in this horrible heat."

Gabriel said, "I have a van full of tools. I've been a mechanic my entire life and always try to be prepared for road emergencies. As you see, there are so few people around and no services for miles and miles."

He pulled his jack out of the van and was able to slip it under the camper. Jacking it up was easy, but getting the rusty bolts off to remove the tire seemed impossible. Sweat ran down into his eyes. The unbearable heat plus the sun baking on his back almost knocked him out. Finally, with a few more big tugs, all the bolts were loose and he pulled the tire off.

"Wow, what a job that was. Now, where's the spare?"

"It's fastened underneath the camper section in a bracket."

Gabriel looked at the low-slung camper and knew he could barely squeeze his bloated body under there. (Too many beers)? He lay on his back in the dirt and inched his way underneath. What he was dreading was exactly what he saw—another set of completely rusted bolts. John handed him the wrench and Gabriel started tugging. He worked with the tire bracket barely above his chest for half an hour. Finally, the last one came loose. As he inched his body out, he was able to reach up and pull the spare out with him.

Designers never seem to think about "how" something was going to be used. It was a simple task if the vehicle was up on a rack in a repair garage with all the hydraulic equipment to loosen bolts. Lying under a vehicle in the dirt was a frustrating challenge.

By that time, Gabriel was seeing stars in his eyes but at least he had the spare. As he took a big breath and shakily stood up, he blinked his eyes and looked again. There was a hole in the tire the size of a grapefruit. It was on the topside of the tire, invisible to him, as he worked so long and hard under the vehicle to loosen it.

He exploded, "What in the hell were you thinking when you took off into this God forsaken wilderness without having your spare tire checked? Don't you know you're endangering the life of your family by being so thoughtless?"

The pained expression on the man's face as he looked at his heat-stricken family was enough. John didn't need any more "chewing out" by a mechanic. As Gabriel saw them standing there with their red faces in the 100-degree heat, he knew he couldn't drive off and leave them.

"John, get in the van with me. I'll take you forward to see what we can find. It shouldn't take long to find a tire; I'll get you right back here and you can be on your way. Your family can stay with the vehicle and run the air for a while as long as the engine doesn't overheat."

He tossed the useless spare in the back of the van and they took off. John's camper was old and the few places they stopped in the next small town didn't have anything that would fit. One of the businesses suggested trying the town ahead that was up and over the next mountain. They looked in the phone book and called every tire shop. Finally they found one that had a tire that would work. However, it was Sunday afternoon; they would be closing in an hour.

"OK, we'll have to try - it's our only chance to find one." Gabriel said. "I have no idea where Patricia is. She must be baking somewhere on the road as I'm way behind her now."

The mountain road was extremely steep. As the van chugged around a corner, Gabriel saw me on the side of the road. I was sitting on my bicycle with my head down on my arms and leaning on the handlebars. I was so hot that I couldn't function anymore. I hardly recognized him. After a brief explanation of his dilemma and my pleading with him not to leave me, Gabriel jumped out of the van and sprayed my clothes with cool water while he tried to figure out what to do. He knew from earlier climbs that my body overheats like a car engine and has to be constantly cooled. He was agonizing about who to leave to expire from the heat and what he could do so nobody died!

If Gabriel slowed to match my snail's pace, it would take at least two hours to make the climb, and then the tire shop would be closed. What was John going to do with his heat-stricken family? The air-conditioner was no longer keeping them cool. If Gabriel took John up over the mountain and back to his family, that would take a couple of hours, and I couldn't hang on that long without him. My only option would be to call the sag and have them pick me up. That would be the end of my goal to pedal every inch of America and the quest for the Guinness Book of Records that Gabriel so dearly wanted for me.

As the moisture evaporated from my wet clothes, my body temperature lowered enough for me to realize that we all were in a serious predicament.

Gabriel said, "Nothing I can do will make this situation work out for everyone. I see the desperation in my wife's eyes. I cannot leave her here on the mountain. We've come a long way, and I need to be by her side. John, I will take you back down where there is phone service and you can try to contact AAA from there."

Gabriel's mind was musing about the sign he had hung in his auto shop: YOUR IGNORANCE DOES NOT CONSTITUTE AN EMERGENCY ON MY BEHALF. He didn't mention it to John because he still had compassion in his heart for his family stuck out in the wasteland.

They turned around to head back down to the corner. Gabriel yelled out his window, "Hang in there Baby, I'll be right back."

When they reached the Mini-Mart location at the bottom, John dialed AAA. "I'm stuck about 60 miles west of Hot Springs. I need help with a flat tire."

"Sir, do you have a spare?"

"I do, but it's no good. It has a hole in it."

"I'm sorry, sir. We can't help you unless you have a spare that is usable. We're not a taxi service." AAA then hung up.

John looked at Gabriel. "Now what do I do?"

Gabriel said, "Let me make a phone call. I've been in this business all my life. I think I can make it happen."

Gabriel dialed, related the problem and got the same response. Then he added, "This gentleman needs help. He's desperate. For a $50 tip, would you consider helping him out?"

"Well, I guess I could. I'm between calls right now."

"The gentleman will be waiting for you at the corner Mini-Mart where the road starts climbing up the mountain."

Gabriel hung up, thrust his fists in the air and shouted, "Yahoo! They'll come."

John shook Gabriel's hand. "How can I ever thank you enough for helping me and my family."

Gabriel jumped in his van, took off up the mountain and found me waiting by the side of the road. My hot, red face sported a big smile as I saw the Love Machine chugging up the hill. Half an hour later, the AAA tow truck, with John in the passenger seat, honked and waved as they passed us on the steep mountain road. We waved back and smiled.

"Gabriel, the Angel" had again lived up to his name!

Day 22:
Hot Springs, SD to
Rapid City, SD

72 miles

Blood oozed out of dozens of tiny fang marks covering my legs. The trickles formed red rivulets running down to stain my white socks. My shoe soles and bicycle tires were covered with black, sticky goo. I had pushed my bike through the tar on the edge of the apron, as I threw it off the road into the drainage ditch. The wheels wouldn't turn because the stones hit the frame and stopped the rotation.

If anyone could have observed the scene on video, I'm pretty sure I looked hilarious. God and Gabriel were the only ones who caught a glimpse of the fiasco. I don't know what God was thinking, but Gabriel was moaning, "What the hell am I doing out here with this crazy woman!"

I was looking forward to the day. As a child growing up in a farming community in Nebraska, taking a trip was a big deal. The Black Hills were almost 400 miles from Swedeburg, Nebraska, population forty-nine. That was five miles outside of Wahoo, a "big town" of 2,000 people.

All four of my grandparents emigrated from Sweden, where they had been farmers. They were in their early twenties when they homesteaded in Nebraska. It was the perfect place to continue doing the only thing they knew how to do. Imagine leaving family and friends, sailing across the Atlantic, crossing half of our huge country, and knowing you would never return home again.

107

Some of my drive and courage must have been inherited from them. Once, as a teenager, along with my Mother and brother, I went to Rapid City to visit my sister and brother-in-law who had recently moved there. The three of us were stylin' as we took off in my brother's black, shiny '49 Oldsmobile 88. I had been awestruck by Mount Rushmore at that time. Who would have thought I would someday ride my bicycle up there?

I had loved cycling around the farm and feeling the wind on my face. The biggest problem was the roads; they were all gravel, dirt or mud. The gravel was the worst; it grabbed my tires and plopped me over. There was never a time in my childhood when I didn't have scabs on my knees and elbows.

Farmers did little traveling beyond day trips, because there were cows to be milked, eggs to be gathered, and animals to be fed. There wasn't anyone else to do it unless it was a real emergency. Then the farmer down the road would try to help in addition to doing his own chores.

All twelve of us in the one-room school that I attended in the 1940's knew about the famous president carvings out of the mountainside in South Dakota's Black Hills. With eight grades in one room, I heard all the lessons every day. I listened to the teacher explain things and watched the older students do their written work on the blackboard so the teacher could see it. By the time I graduated from eighth grade, I was pretty smart – at least I thought so.

After pedaling 106 and 120 miles into the wind in Wyoming, a 72-mile day should have been a breeze. Every day was unique, and that day we had to factor in 100-degree heat plus humidity with almost the same numbers. An additional challenge of the day was a nine-mile climb up to Mount Rushmore with a ten percent grade (a clone of our local Gibraltar Road) plus another 5,400 feet of climbing along the way.

The winding uphill roads led us into the Black Hills National Forest. Cars, buses and trucks heading up to the famous four whizzed by; but at least there was a shoulder to ride on. Although the heat was oppressive and already into the nineties, I pedaled the climbs without too much difficulty. I thought the day might not be so hard after all. I should have known better.

Suddenly the wide road ended. Construction signs everywhere warned roadwork was being done on the last, extremely steep section of road leading up to the top of the mountain. I had been climbing all morning; I was so hot, how was I going to get up to Mount Rushmore?

Gabriel had caught up but didn't even try to stay by me. As I started rounding curves and climbing, there were no turnouts, not even for a bicycle. What next? Narrow road – fresh tar – horse flies – blood – dancing on the roadway?

Santa Barbara occasionally has a little tar on the beaches; people fret over a blob the size of a dime. My shoes and all the crevices in the soles were covered with tar. Every inch of sole space had rocks stuck to it. I was the abominable snowman with heavy shoes I could hardly lift.

When Gabriel and the Love Machine chugged up the mountain a few minutes later, he kept going until he found a spot to pull over and then ran back down to where I was.

He had thought I was really nuts when he came around the corner and saw me dancing and jumping up and down in the middle of the road. He didn't know I had been attacked by a swarm of horseflies, and they were biting me all over. There were at least several dozen bites on my legs that each left two little fang marks.

I was wearing shorts and a long sleeved shirt; my body had some protection, but not my legs. When Gabriel got to me and saw my bleeding legs, he sprinted back to the van and grabbed the water spray bottle and a towel. He started wetting my legs and wiping off the blood. The flies had bitten through the Hanes hosiery I always wore.

Gabriel was aghast. Those were the legs he loved. His former female friends were short and had stubby legs. One of the first things he had noticed about me was my long, slim legs.

Was I ever a mess! I was already sticky and hot and sweaty from pumping up the long, steep hill. As I frantically hopped around, I hadn't noticed where I was jumping. With the extreme heat, the tar on the side of the road was melted goo.

"Road Under Construction" signs were everywhere. I had tried to be careful, as I climbed up the mountain, to stay on the road itself and keep out of the tiny apron on the side. The fresh tar had collected there as the machines packed the stones into the roadway and squeezed it to the side.

Gabriel started working on my shoes to get the stones off. They wouldn't stay off until the tar was out of all the cracks on the soles. Bicycle shoes have many cracks to give good traction on the pedals. My pubic bone would be screaming if my foot slipped off the pedal towards the ground.

There wasn't even any place to sit down to take my shoes off as everything was "gooey." Good thing there wasn't much traffic.

When the horse flies started swarming on me, I instinctively tried to get away from them. Because the hill was so steep, and I was having difficulty pushing the pedals around, I couldn't ride away. In my frenzy, I tossed my bike in the ditch. I didn't want to leave it on the road to be run over by a car or truck.

I was basically a free meal for those hungry little critters. Many times during the ride I had cried in frustration, but that time I was laughing, as the whole scene was so ridiculous.

When I heard the buzzing of a swarm, my first thought was bees. My mother was deathly afraid of bees and wasps and for good reason. She got stung in our yard while pulling weeds.

110

The neighbor saw her lying motionless on the ground and rushed her into town. The doctor said she had an allergic reaction to the stings. Because she had lost consciousness, if she were ever to be stung again, she probably would have died.

Knowing that from my childhood, I, too, was afraid of bees and wasps, fearing I may have the same biological tendencies as my mother. The swarming sound panicked me and sent my adrenalin soaring. I wasn't thinking about something as mundane as staying out of the tar.

I was lucky. It was horse flies instead of bees or wasps that decided to lunch on my tasty legs. After a stern admonition from Gabriel, "Don't you dare get into that melted tar strip again," I gingerly started climbing. The tar-studded road that climbed for a total of nine miles was another one of those "eternal climbs."

When cars honked at me to get over, I kept my head down, held my space and kept slowly pushing those pedals around. Many drivers were considerate of cyclists; but there were others who thought they owned the entire road, and the cyclist should be riding in the ditch. No one could see my thoroughly bitten and bloody legs to understand why I really didn't want to deal with the goo again.

The scenery was magnificent. The Black Hills were so dense that everywhere I looked, it was breathtaking. I understood how they got their name – the trees were so big and thick, they looked more black than green.

When the treacherous road ended, it joined one that was a little more reasonable. We still had climbing to do, but at least we had a shoulder to ride on.

The first carving I saw was on the right, Crazy Horse Monument. Many signs enticed us to stop at their museum and look around. After the morning workout I had conquered, I was ready.

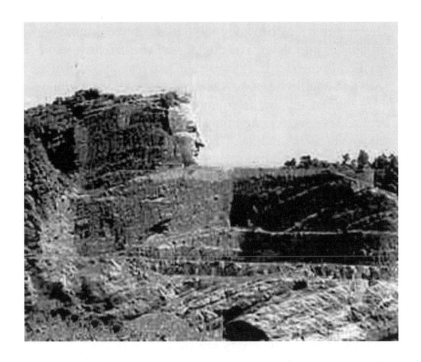

We parked down below; Gabriel unloaded his bike, and we pedaled the mile up to the museum together. He was huffing and puffing when we got to the top.

He was always muttering, "I don't understand how you do it."

The close-up look of Crazy Horse Monument was so cool. We spent a couple of hours there enjoying the museum and talking with people. Their response was always, "You're doing what?" Gabriel loved to tell them I was 67 years old and watch their jaws drop!

After riding down from Crazy Horse, Gabriel attached his bike to the back of the van again. A few miles further up the road, we started getting glimpses of the back of someone's head on Mount Rushmore.

Earlier we had viewed the faces from afar. Now it was awesome to be next to them. I understood why people came from all over the world to Mount Rushmore. It was mind-boggling how those faces could have been carved and chiseled out of a mountain.

As I rounded the last curve to pull in front of the faces, I was appalled to see a huge, tiered parking structure. Was I dreaming? Was I back in Los Angeles? You either had to pay to enter the huge piece of cement that funneled you into the museum or take off down the road to Rapid City. We were glad we had stopped at Crazy Horse.

We did a "no-no" and pulled over on the shoulder to take our pictures. The huge blob of concrete didn't compliment God's beauty that I had been lapping up all morning.

Tom, our computer guru expert in Santa Barbara, had made a fabulous tongue-in-cheek portrait of Mount Rushmore's four men and ME, a woman peeking out from between them.

Tom's caption "There needs to be a woman on Mt. Rushmore – so why not Patricia" had our friends chuckling. Clever Tom kept the website updated every day while we were traipsing across the country.

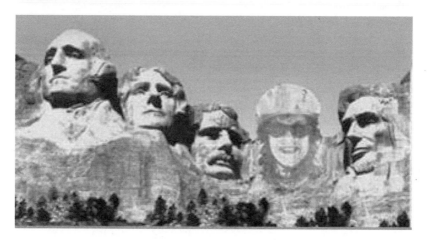

And then, I had the most wonderful downhill ride. When I got down the mountain on the north side, it was time to do some climbing again to get into Rapid City.

That night at dinner, Gabriel had fun talking about his dancing wife and her episode with the horse flies. Everyone was laughing; but I was thinking it's one of those things you needed to be there to get the whole picture.

Sometimes it's better to laugh than cry, and that day was my chance to laugh at myself.

Day 23:
Rapid City, SD to
Wall, SD

57 miles

Outside of Rapid City, we cycled through The
Badlands, an area of unusual combinations of chiseled peaks,
rugged ridges, canyons and prairie. Wall is a tourist town of
around 800 residents that boasts of one thousand motel rooms.
Many places we have traveled through are closed during the
cold winter months. How do they manage to survive and pay
the bills?

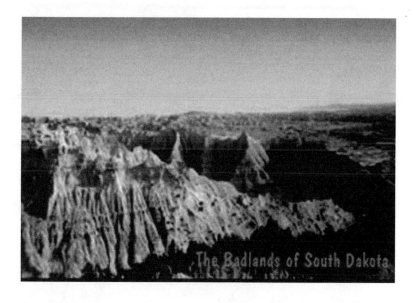

There really was a natural wall, a strip several miles
wide and nine miles long of spires, ridges and twisted gullies

that divided the prairie area. Thus the nearby town got its name of Wall, South Dakota.

Talk about gullible. Someone had told me the town was famous because the family that started Wal-Mart was from the area and I had passed the news along. When we got into town, I found out it was not true – how embarrassing!

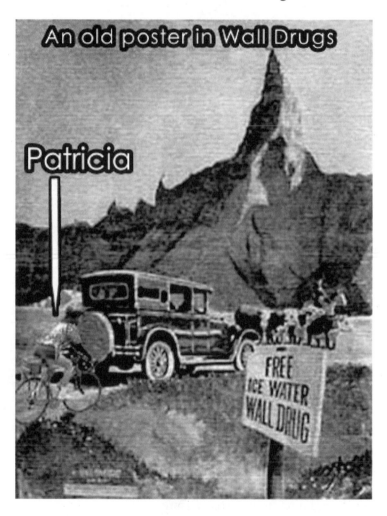

An old poster in Wall Drugs

Patricia

The short day was welcome as the next day was expected to be a lulu. We had to get up at 4:30 a.m. and rain was forecast to add to the heat and headwinds. Hang on Patricia!

Day 24:
Wall, SD to Pierre, SD
117 miles

On a map of the United States, South Dakota is directly above Nebraska. It was a challenge every day to keep my mind full without external stimulation. For safety reasons, no one rode with earphones. It was necessary to be tuned in at all times to my surroundings. There might be only one vehicle every ten or fifteen minutes, but I needed to know exactly where it was in the landscape, or it could wipe me off the face of the earth.

I was reminded of memories from high school in Wahoo, Nebraska where I played the lead in a Willa Cather play about western Nebraska. The character described the loneliness and isolation associated with the barren wilderness. I recalled learning and delivering a five-page soliloquy where the heroine went crazy. Now I understood the depth of feeling that pushed her to that point. The only difference was that I experienced the feeling each day on my bicycle and had the ability to move on. She couldn't; and it was more than she could handle mentally.

That thought kept me pedaling during the hot, grueling, extremely long day into the wind. We were only a few days from Mitchell, the purported "Corn Capitol" of the world.

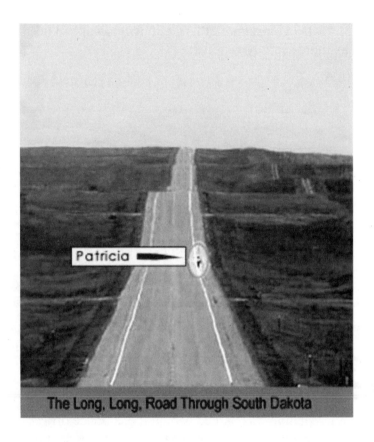

The Long, Long, Road Through South Dakota

I needed a cornfield! It signified life and security to this stubborn Cornhusker who was challenging every part of her being. Pedaling alone in nature's desolation or surrounded with growing green was not the same. Mentally, I had gone as far as I could go.

Do you suppose this Cottonwood jail had been their maximum-security facility?

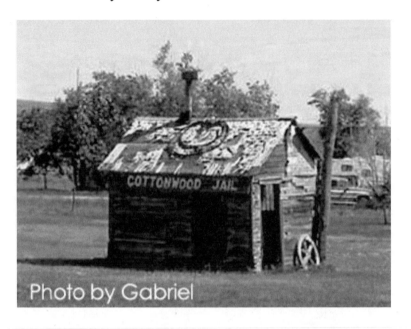

Photo by Gabriel

At one turnout in the road where I was snacking and the Love Machine was parked behind me, a police officer pulled up and stopped to ask if we were okay. When we told him what I was attempting and my age, I think he thought I was a little tetched in the head for being out there in such miserable conditions. I knew he was right, but that didn't stop me.

Gabriel stayed closer to Bill and me, my back end buddy who was around somewhere, so he could help soothe us with the cold water bottles he pulled out of his cooler.

The seemingly endless day translated to 13 ½ hours on my bicycle. The nice patrolman probably knew what he was talking about. One consoling thought was that I would pass over the halfway mark somewhere tomorrow. I had no thought of abandoning my crazy dream.

DAY 25:
PIERRE, SD TO
CHAMBERLAIN, SD

84 MILES

Heat and wind – what else should I have expected on the prairie in July. The locals said it was 108 degrees last year – we should feel lucky it was only 102. I found out at breakfast that even the "big guys" were struggling yesterday. "Little twiggy me" wasn't the only one suffering.

For the first 35 miles we were once again dealing with the unbearable wind. Then it disappeared as we rode along the Missouri River for the first time. I remembered the "muddy Mo" from my childhood as it flowed by Omaha, Nebraska. How different it looked here in South Dakota without the mud. It was shades of blue and green with the sun sparkling and shimmering off the water.

Gabriel found me at the second rest stop about 1:30 p.m. and started wetting me down. I couldn't have survived the intense heat without him. I felt like a droopy, wilted plant.

Water meant trees and greenery as we approached the scenic town of Chamberlain, nestled up to the river.

When it was time for dinner, Gabriel wasn't in our room. I found him in the van.

"Hi, Baby, aren't you cooking out here when you could be in our air conditioned room?"

"I'm okay. I'm cleaning house."

"C'mon, let's go to dinner. I'm starved as usual."

"Just let me finish my soda. Start walking over and I'll catch up with you."

"Okay, but please come soon."

I waited in the cool entrance to the restaurant about five minutes until Gabriel showed up. When we went in, I walked over to a long table where seven or eight of our cyclists were sitting.

"Let's sit here."

"I don't want to sit with anyone else tonight."

"Oh, come on. I don't want them to think we're stuck up."

I pulled out a chair and sat down and Gabriel followed suit by sitting as far away from anyone as possible. He was glaring at me, but I tried to ignore it. I didn't know what was wrong, but didn't want to make any kind of a scene in front of our friends. We ate with little conversation between us and as soon as we finished, Gabriel said, "Let's get out of here."

I said "Goodbye, see you tomorrow a.m." to everyone and followed Gabriel out of the restaurant. He didn't stop to talk to anyone.

When we got outside, he started in on me, "Don't you ever do that again."

"Do what again, I didn't do anything but you sure were rude to everyone at dinner."

"When I say I want to be alone, I mean it. I didn't want to sit with anyone else."

I then realized my suspicions were true. He was drinking more than soda in the van and he knew it was going to hit him. The extreme heat was adding to the alcohol's intensification. It was a miracle he only drank after we reached our destination – never while driving.

I knew the writing was on the wall. When we got back to our room, he wouldn't stop talking and taking digs at me.

"I told you in Santa Barbara I didn't want to come on this stupid adventure. You're not going to make it across the country so why don't you quit now. Let's go home."

"Are you crazy? Did you forget I made it over the Continental Divide a few days ago and now you're telling me to quit? No way. If you'd rather go home and drink, go back to Santa Barbara and I'll go on alone. I'll miss you like crazy but I'll figure it out. Nothing is going to stop me – certainly not your drinking." I went into the bathroom, slammed the door and took a long relaxing bath. By the time I got out, Gabriel was passed out in bed – thank God. I didn't have any energy left to deal with alcohol.

Day 26:
Chamberlain, SD to
Mitchell, SD

70 miles

"Gabriel, who was the shapely gal that whizzed by on the bicycle and waved? It certainly can't be your 67 year old wife!"

"Yes, Amy Dee, it was. I told you, she's hot. Nobody believes her age. On top of that, she's pedaling that damn bicycle all the way across America. My foot is sore from pushing on the gas pedal, and I'm exhausted at the end of each day after watching her struggle up all those mountains – I'm only teasing. I haven't figured out where she gets her stamina."

"Gabriel, my daughters, Kristine and Sophia, and I were headed out of town with a full schedule planned for today; but, after meeting you and getting a glimpse of your wife, I'm canceling everything. I want to meet Patricia. Why is she doing this—there must be a reason to survive all the punishment Mother Nature can dish out?"

"Patricia is a musician pedaling for our local City College. She's determined to raise $22,000 so she can have a perpetual scholarship awarded every year with her name on it."

Amy Dee continued, "The mayor of Mitchell is a friend of mine, as I've worked on several of her committees. I'm getting on the phone right now to arrange for us to meet for dinner tonight. The mayor is in her 70's and a real pistol. She has been so successful in making our town thrive. She would love to meet Patricia. I'm going to make it happen. Here's my phone number. Call me when Patricia gets into Mitchell and I'll tell you where to meet us."

"Amy Dee, this is awesome. I was sitting here at the intersection waiting for Patricia to pedal by, and you drove up asking *me* for directions. That was really funny, as I've been continually lost since I left Santa Barbara. I know Patricia will be excited to meet the mayor and you and your family. I should be calling you between five and six tonight. Bye for now."

It was a relatively short day with seventy plus miles to pedal, but the ferocious wind never stopped. I felt like the "little twig" again being battered around and was thankful the twig hadn't snapped in two. Gabriel caught up with me in early afternoon.

"Baby, I'm really excited. At an intersection ten miles back down the road, I met this great gal and her two pretty daughters. They saw me parked and pulled up behind to ask for directions. When they realized I couldn't help them, the mother started asking questions about you. They had been looking at the signs on the Love Machine. Amy Dee could hardly believe her eyes when you pedaled by. She said she knows the mayor of Mitchell and will arrange a dinner for this evening. She also said the Mayor will give you the key to the city."

"Sure sounds like a fairytale to me; having dinner with the mayor and getting a key to a city? Are you already drinking this early in the day?"

"I'm not teasing and I'm not sauced," Gabriel retorted. "Amy Dee said she could arrange the meeting so we'll see what happens. Maybe *she's* smoking something. We'll find out when we get in to town."

Gabriel got into Mitchell before I did. When I finally blew in, he started dialing Amy Dee. Sure, having dinner with the mayor and getting a key from someone's promise at an intersection, I might as well soak my aching body in the bathtub for an hour or two.

Just as I sank into the warm, soothing water, Gabriel started banging on the bathroom door.

"Baby, hurry up. Get out and get dressed. Amy Dee said we should be at a restaurant a few blocks from here in thirty minutes. Mayor Alice will be there."

Sure. This sounds like a hoax. I'd rather soak.

More bangs on the door. "Come on, baby, please get out of there and get ready."

Guess I should humor him. He really is a nice guy to be rolling across the country with me.

When we walked into the restaurant, Mayor Alice was waiting for us. Amy Dee and her daughters showed up a few minutes later.

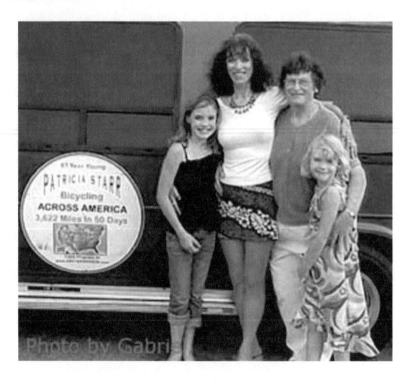

The Mayor was everything Amy Dee had mentioned to Gabriel. She was a warm, genuinely caring Midwesterner. She gave both of us big hugs and welcomed us to Mitchell.

What a woman. Alice had been directing the town of Mitchell for three terms as mayor. Her town of less than 15,000 residents boasted 19 parks, two golf courses, a recreation center with indoor pool; basketball and racquetball courts; one baseball diamond and fourteen softball diamonds; five soccer fields; a skating and ice hockey arena; a twenty-four lane bowling alley and Lake Mitchell to provide boating, swimming and fishing. She had obtained five million dollars in federal grants to be spent on much needed water projects. Whew! She was one busy lady!

After dinner, Kristine, the twelve-year-old daughter, interviewed me for a school project. Then Mayor Alice presented me with the key to the city of Mitchell, an unprecedented thrill.

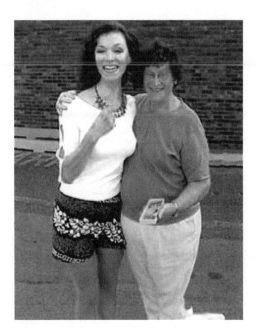

She said, "Patricia, it was such an honor to spend the evening with a woman who has so many dreams and is accomplishing them. I am in awe of what you are doing – pedaling America and endowing scholarships."

I replied, "Mayor Alice, we are both women who are turning our dreams into reality. The ride across America was never about pushing the pedals around. It is the adventures along the way and the people we meet. You have made me feel like a queen. You will be an inspiration to me and to every other life you touch. Your accomplishments in Mitchell will never be forgotten."

We truly had a mutual admiration society.

It was difficult to say goodbye to those wonderful people; but it had been a long day, and we wanted to get to the Corn Palace before it closed.

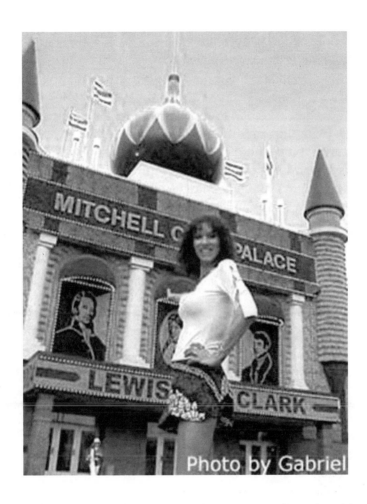

Photo by Gabriel

In Nebraska, many knew of the Corn Palace, but I had never been there. My mind had pictured it as an Indian tepee. What a surprise! It looked like Las Vegas or Disneyland, an incredible work of art and a museum combined in one. It was difficult to comprehend how corncobs and cornhusks could be so decorative. The Palace was built in 1892 to show the world that South Dakota had a healthy agricultural climate. The first two buildings were outgrown, and the present one was

129

completed in 1921. In the thirties, kiosks and minarets of
Moorish design were added on.

The Corn Palace is a multi-festival building used for
exhibits, dances, stage shows, proms, graduations, and
statewide basketball tournaments. It gets redecorated every
year with thirteen different colors of corn, grain, and native
grasses to make it the "agricultural showplace of the world."
Ear by ear, the corn is painstakingly nailed to the Corn Palace
which enjoys 50,000 visitors from around the world each year.
Remember, this is in the middle of nowhere.

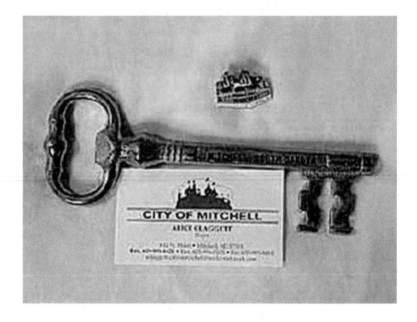

Was I excited to get a key to the city of Mitchell?
It was an honor I will never forget!

Day 27:
Mitchell, SD to
Sioux Falls, SD

72 miles

Mayor Alice was the epitome of mid-western hospitality. I'm pedaling away to be an inspiration to others to get out and do something—whatever that may happen to be. Don't be concerned about the age number on your driver's license.

Last night we met the perfect example of one woman who has made a difference—not only in her community, but in the lives of so many around her.

She was planning to jump off the diving board in a 20's costume when the new pool was dedicated. Wish I could have been there to cheer her on and applaud. She's my kind of woman.

The day was overcast so we had a welcome break from the intense heat. My legs were spinning fast now that I was the proud recipient of the key to the city of Mitchell – what an honor. Then Gabriel took a phone call from Tom saying that Bob and Mary Elliot of Santa Barbara had pledged 25 cents a mile to my scholarship fund, so my legs were really flying We were so happy and thankful for every donation, whatever the size, as they all helped our goal of placing the scholarship into perpetuity!

Cycling into Sioux Falls was no picnic. We had been in the boonies for so long that we had forgotten about the traffic tribulations within a city. We finally made it to the motel and did a quick turnaround, as we had an interview with the local TV station KELO. I was part of the news that evening and also the next day. That was always exciting.

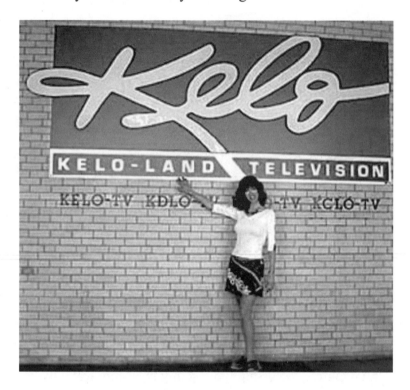

Tomorrow would be a long-awaited rest day. I even had a glass of wine with my dinner because of the day off. Some of the cyclists imbibed daily, but with my delicate body balance and goal to pedal every inch, I wasn't taking any chances. I needed to be at peak performance every hour of the day.

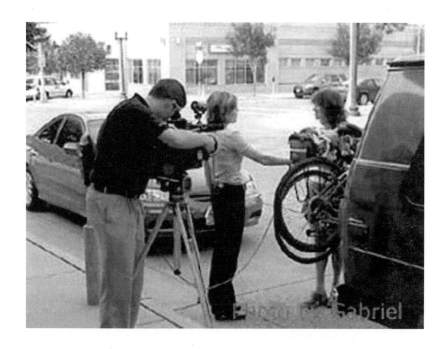

Day 28:
Rest Day in
Sioux Falls, SD

We went shopping! How could something so ordinary be such a big deal? After fighting my way across the loneliness, heat and wind of South Dakota, my soul needed a little massaging. I was the lucky one – we had our Love Machine to do some sightseeing and then stopped at the most fabulous Sporting Goods store imaginable. Everything to do with sports was sold under one roof. It was called Cabela's; a chain scattered across the country, although not in the Santa Barbara area. It was a huge, multi-story building that soared all the way to the top in the center; but, the various floors looked out on to the atrium that contained huge palm trees.

Those Midwesterners know how to give a structure some ambiance.

We had taken care of necessary computer work and laundry in the morning. The remainder of the day brought me back to earth to prepare for conquering the next step in my dream.

Day 29: Sioux Falls, SD to Worthington, MN

65 miles

The day started with an intensely green bicycle trail. I could imagine I was riding on the famous Pebble Beach Golf Course in California. A twenty-mile loop of manicured grass on both sides of the path circled the entire city and seemed to roll on forever. We rode ten miles of the trail as we exited Sioux Falls.

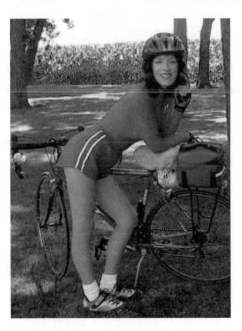

It was mind-boggling to think the state of South Dakota had made something so beautiful that could be enjoyed only half the year because of the extreme weather. This was the same state that made the thoughtless rumble bumps directly on the shoulder strip so we had nowhere to ride.

The glorious beginning almost made me forget the crummy detour we hit right after the bike path ended. We rode miles and miles on a dusty gravel road.

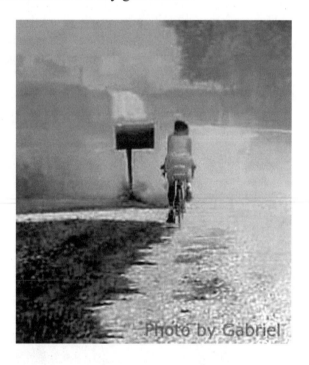

Memories of skinned knees as a kid had to be squelched so I could pay attention and not slip.

Gabriel had pictures of a cute dog chasing me down the gravel road. Tom, our computer guru, had captioned the photos on the website: *Then along the way a new friend comes to greet you and protect you from the weird guy in the blue van. The*

136

four-footed friend tags along for a way before going back to sleep under the porch. Patricia made his day!

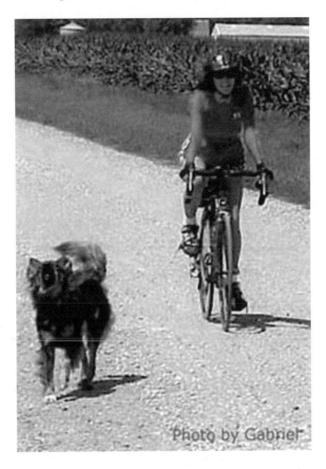

Photo by Gabriel

   Twenty-four miles into the ride I crossed into Minnesota, the fifth state on the itinerary. Luckily, Minnesota's famous giant mosquitoes hadn't yet discovered how tasty I was.

Day 30:
Worthington, MN to
Mankato, MN

102 miles

There was definitely a "new look" as we pedaled along with cornfields on all sides. The buildings were all well-kept, neatly painted and in good repair. Gone were the picturesque, collapsing barns of South Dakota.

We had two back-to-back centuries as we started our travels across Minnesota. The riding was relatively flat and much appreciated.

People everywhere were friendly. I had pulled over for a snack, and a couple of bicyclists stopped. They were not from our group, but were training for "the big one" across Iowa (10,000 cyclists). They had done the ride several times and talked about the special camaraderie that existed. That's a mind-boggling number of pedalers to be passing through any state. They mentioned that some of the thoughtful farmers had left rolls of toilet paper on their fence posts. Mother Nature, at times, can't be ignored.

Rain was on the way. When Gabriel caught up to me in mid-afternoon, I ate my special "beans and weenies" lunch sitting in the van while the shower passed over. Then it became extremely hot and sticky – mid-westerners knew the feeling when temperature and humidity shoot upward at the same time.

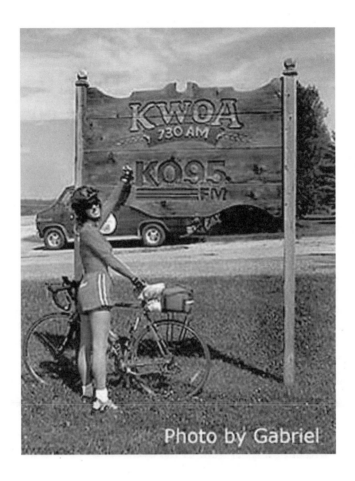

Photo by Gabriel

As we rolled into Mankato, we stopped at radio station KWOA, KO95 for an interview. The personnel were always amazed at the feat and happy to talk to us. I've pedaled over 2,000 miles—who would have dreamed...

Day 31: Mankato, MN to Rochester, MN

101 miles

What a bizarre day...

Gabriel was rolling down the highway about seventy mph. After half a mile, he felt, oh-no!—thumpety, thumpety, thump, thump, thump, and the van pulling hard to the right. It was that awful feeling most of us have experienced, a flat tire. He pulled onto the shoulder and got out to see the damage.

He walked around the front of the van to inspect the offending front tire and said a few choice words. He knew Duane and I were waiting for him in the next town. At least he had a spare, and being the good mechanic he is, he knew it had air in it. As he walked to the rear to get the spare off the back door, he heard a hissing sound. He looked down to see the right rear tire deflating in front of his eyes.

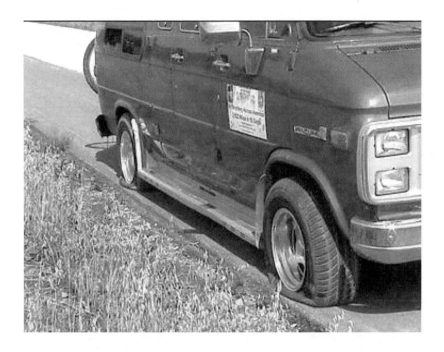

"Damn it! This can't be happening to me."

Whatever punctured the front tire must have been firmly lodged in the road and subsequently punctured the back one too. Even my mechanically inclined husband couldn't solve that problem with only one spare.

He tried to get me on the phone to tell me what had happened, but I was too far ahead. I had been on the road since six o'clock that morning. I planned to meet a friend from Santa Barbara who played in the Prime Time Band. I had known Duane for many years, but had not seen him for a while. When I arrived for my first rehearsal three years ago, he was playing trumpet in the band.

Duane was going to be visiting relatives in July. After comparing notes, we realized we would be at almost the same place at the same time. His family home was only about five miles from Medford. I told him the date and approximate time I would be riding through town, and he said he would be there to meet me.

Boogie'n down the road, I had gone almost fifty miles by 11:30, the agreed time for Duane and me to meet. As I rolled down the street on the outskirts of town, I saw Duane standing on the sidewalk by a neat little white house. He had found a good parking place under a big tree.

The temperature was very Midwestern: hot and humid. The thermometer on the downtown corner bank building had already hit 90 degrees.

After some good hugs, Duane asked, "What's it really feel like pedaling all those miles?"

I responded, "If you got up every day for forty-five days and knew you had to cycle from Santa Barbara to either Los Angeles or Disneyland, that's what it feels like. It's a heck of a long way, even in a car!"

We sat on the sidewalk and chatted for almost an hour. "Duane, this has been fabulous. You are the first tie to home in many weeks, but I still have a long way to go. I apologize for Gabriel's not showing up. He knew about our meeting here."

I tried dialing Gabriel again but no connection.

I hugged Duane and said, "Please tell everyone back in Santa Barbara 'hello' from me."

As I started out of town, my mind was still nagging, *where was Gabriel?* He never was good at keeping time. He had intentions, but got lost in the moment of whatever he happened to be doing. I've waited for him and done a little fuming of my own on many occasions. It's an idiosyncrasy with which I've learned to live.

I still had fifty plus miles to go, and I was already boiling hot and sweaty. After I pedaled about an hour, my phone rang. I pulled over quickly.

It was Gabriel. "You're not going to believe what happened to me today and where I am."

My first question was, "Are you OK?"

142

"Yes, but I sure had a problem this morning."

He knew about our rendezvous with Duane around lunchtime, so he had hurried and left the motel earlier than usual. About ten miles out of Mankato, he got a call from a newspaper reporter who was writing an article about me in the local press. He pulled onto the shoulder so he could talk and take notes if necessary. It had been raining earlier; the shoulder was soft and slippery, but Gabriel was able to ease the van off the road.

They had a great conversation about the bicycle ride, my age, and what a challenge every single day was. Gabriel started the van and began to pull onto the road. The wheels were spinning in the mud, but he gunned it and got into the traffic flow. He looked at his watch. He's a great talker; he knew he was cutting the timing pretty close.

"Baby, that's the wildest thing that's ever happened to me in a car. I had two flat tires at once, and I was stuck out in the middle of nowhere. I was so disgusted and felt so helpless. I not only missed lunch with you and Duane, I know this is a long, hot day and I wanted to be there to help you. I was able to contact a tow truck in Mankato, the town where we just spent the night."

Now my private afternoon sag wagon was waiting to be "sagged." What an irony!

When the tow truck finally arrived, the driver and Gabriel decided to tow it to the little town of Owatonna, the biggest place around. It was a few miles from where Duane and I were meeting; not on the same road to Medford, but off the route to the south.

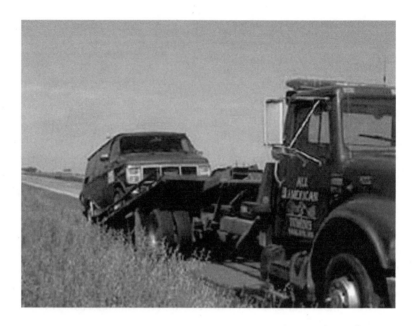

It shouldn't be difficult to buy two tires. But in that small town, no one had a special-sized pair. Gabriel kept walking from shop to shop. He finally found two that would do and had them delivered to the shop where the van was waiting.

In the meantime, the town was having a special celebration day. The Wells Fargo Bank was putting on lunch for anyone who wanted to come. Gabriel was hungry so he stopped in. He was impressed with the bank building and the murals covering the walls. It was one of the original banks along the trail of the wagon trains, as they came through Minnesota. It had been designated as an architectural landmark.

After lunch, he walked through the small park adjacent to the bank. Two sidewalks intersected, and the gentleman on the other sidewalk started talking with him. They conversed about the bank building and the charm of the small town. The other man continued, "My jewelry store is across the street. Stop on by."

Gabriel had nothing to occupy his time, so he went into the store. He knew it would be a while before the Love Machine was ready for the road again. It was lunchtime for everyone, and in those small towns, you just had to wait.

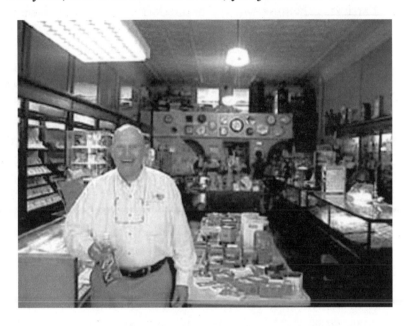

Gabriel explained to the jeweler. "I'm here because of some rotten luck, two flat tires at once. My wife is pedaling across America, and I'm already late for lunch with her and a special friend. She's going to be so ticked off at me."

The jeweler looked at him, "I know all about your wife and her trip across America. You must be Gabriel."

Gabriel's mouth dropped in disbelief. He was speechless. How could he meet someone in the middle of Minnesota who knew him by name?

Gabriel's mind was tumbling: *What's going on here? Am I in the middle of a Sci-Fi movie? Does this guy have ESP? Has the vodka I've been nipping after Patricia passes out at night destroyed my brain cells? Did I really hear someone call me by my name, Gabriel?*

The jeweler spoke again, "The man your wife met before lunch is my best friend, Duane. He told me all about Patricia. When you walked in the door and said your wife was pedaling America, bingo! I knew you must be Gabriel."

Gabriel responded, "Wow, you're making me feel better. I really thought I was losing it. You didn't know me when we chatted outside in the park. I can't begin to tell you how weird I felt. I'm a Santa Barbara native, so when I'm home, many people know me. I've been on the road now for over five weeks, and nobody knows me. Then I walk into a jewelry store, and someone calls me Gabriel. Talk about a strange coincidence. I've never had two flat tires at the same time before, and I end up in a town that isn't even on the route across America. How did I start the day on the freeway and meet the best friend of the man we were to meet before lunch, because two sidewalks intersected? The chances of that happening must be about the same odds as winning the lottery."

It was a long, slow process to get both tires delivered, changed, and the Love Machine ready to hit the road again. Gabriel was able to get through to me and tell me where he was and what had happened; and that he didn't miss the visit with Duane because "he forgot." Before I got Gabriel's phone call, I had pedaled out of town without getting anything to eat. I thought he was coming soon with lunch for us.

It didn't take long to realize I was going to be in big trouble that afternoon. It was now after two o'clock. I couldn't think of pedaling all the way back to get food. Hopefully, my husband would get to me soon.

The 90 degrees registered on the bank thermometer before noon was only the beginning.

The hills got steeper; the temperature got hotter; I got weaker. My blood sugar dropped fast; I felt my coordination coming unglued. My mind was no longer sharp. My concentration was gone. My stomach was churning and nauseated. I had lost touch with reality. I'd been there before. I knew the feelings.

How could I continue to ride with all this going wrong inside my body? I was having my own flat tires. I was alone and the fear of not knowing what was going to happen to me flooded through me.

I looked up and couldn't believe what I saw in front of me. Most of the hills today had been pretty manageable, but now I saw this long, long climb ahead.

I pulled over to get a drink of water. At least I had some with me; but it, too, was hot. I could have sat down on the shoulder and cried, but that wouldn't solve anything. I kept staring at the long hill with the blazing sun beating on it. How could I possibly climb it feeling like I did?

As I sat by the road, my guardian angel must have felt the distress I was in. I watched in amazement as four little clouds appeared overhead. The rest of the sky was blue and clear. The clouds gave a bit of shade to take the burning sun off of me.

Then the most astonishing thing happened. The clouds started moving their spot of shade up the long, long, hill. I hopped back on my bicycle and started pedaling. I was able to stay in their shade all the way to the top. The blistering sun couldn't touch me.

It was incredible.

By now it was almost four o'clock. As I rode over the crest of the long climb, I saw that Bill, on the recumbent bike, had pulled over to rest a few minutes. The hill had been torture for him, too.

"Bill," I babbled. "I don't think I can go on. I'm so hot, and my blood sugar has dropped out of sight. My angel sent some clouds to help me get up the last hill."

Bill must have thought I'd gone over the edge.

147

I babbled on, "Gabriel called me a couple of hours ago. He had two flat tires, but I need him now."

Bill immediately dialed Gabriel, but there was no connection. He understood how fragile I was and suggested we ride together. He didn't like anyone following him closely, but knew I desperately needed a lifeline. We rode that way for the next hour.

At five o'clock my phone rang. It was Gabriel. He said, "I finally have the van on the road and I'm trying to find you. I'm completely lost because the town where I was towed isn't on our bicycle route map. I'm so frustrated, and I know I'm letting you down. This whole flat tire situation sucks. Baby, look at your map; and help me find where the hell I am."

I dug my map out of my bag. I was so far gone, mentally, I couldn't function. I handed the map and phone to Bill and begged, "Please, help me. I'm so incoherent, I don't even know where I am."

Bill was able to communicate to Gabriel where we were. Then we hit the road again. Fifteen minutes later, I heard the purring of the Love Machine. My lunch had arrived. What a feast! I was like the energizer bunny that wound up when you fed me. That was the closest I had been to total body collapse.

We thanked Bill many times for being there for me when I was ready to check out. Gabriel always had a cold bottle of water for Bill, and he so appreciated it.

Bill took off down the road while I woofed down my five o'clock lunch. Gabriel filled me in on the happenings during his bizarre day. What a strange coincidence that Gabriel met the jeweler. I wish I could have met him too. He sounded like a really nice guy.

The big city of Rochester, home of the famous Mayo Clinic, was still an hour away. I never would have been able to cope with the rush hour traffic in the city without my lunch.

I wheeled into the motel, thanking my angels—Bill, Gabriel and my guardian angel for helping me survive another day.

Day 32:
Rochester, MN to
LaCrosse, WI

89 miles

If all the male bicyclists pedaling America were in a line-up, the one I'd pick as the "hunk" of the group and in the best physical shape was now imprisoned in the sag wagon. He was a handsome doctor, probably mid-40's, a kidney transplant surgeon from the San Francisco Bay area in California. He was one of the three "buddies" from med school reuniting to pedal America.

Biking into Rochester yesterday, he was experiencing extreme pain and swelling in the thigh area of one leg. Nothing traumatic like an accident or collision had triggered the problem. The timing was perfect as he was at the world-famous Mayo Clinic. Because of his position as a doctor, he didn't have a problem getting an appointment for an MRI.

The prognosis was as expected – rest and pain pills. After all the anticipation of riding America, how disappointing to end up in the sag wagon. You're still "there" but have to experience the daily trek from an entirely different perspective. The hundred plus miles must be boring considering you are trapped in the wagon for the entire day.

How scary when I heard what had happened to the handsome doc. That could have been me. My dream to pedal America would be shattered. The group wouldn't wait for an injury to heal. The sag wagon would be the only option. My strength and experience are miniscule in comparison to a well-trained body. None of us are immune to injuries.

I surely did have to work hard to pedal the distance each day and sometimes it was excruciating. I'm grateful my body was holding up except for my nagging broken toe. Fatigue was fixable. The doc's leg wasn't. His original diagnosis prescribed a day-by-day evaluation of his condition. In other words, let nature handle it.

After completing back-to-back centuries, an easy day would have been welcome. Bicyclists talked with pride about their centuries. I never had one before. By the end of the ride, I would have done at least eight, maybe more. Some of the days that had ninety plus miles on paper could also be over a hundred, counting detours we had to take (no choice) and the times I had been lost (my fault).

I rode alone until early or mid-afternoon and had to make decisions on my own. Sometimes, I goofed.

Our maps were guidelines. The different roads we encountered were not always marked. Many times it was a guess. My odometer was new when I left Santa Barbara. It was not working correctly, and no one seemed to be able to fix it – not even the bicycle shops we had visited on our days off. It registered the number of miles, but would not turn back to zero.

At this point, my odometer read 2,175 miles. It was difficult to add the numbers on the sheet and keep them in my head, while I pedaled along trying to keep my body going and hoping not to be annihilated by cars and trucks.

The mileage on the map said 89 miles but we had only pedaled a few miles before we saw the dreaded "DETOUR" signs. Our road maps were developed and printed many months ago, so we never had advance notice of road closures. We were able to worm our way through the construction on the first detour; but when we approached the second one, everything was completely closed off. We had to go back and start over. The extra miles pushed us to extra centuries.

151

The only other road available was composed of extremely steep rollers. The four guys that let me tag along were my friends. I pedaled all the hills, as they patiently waited for me to come over the crest before they took off on the next roller. It was a struggle. Without them, I would have been completely lost out in the country – alone again. Once off the beaten path, no one knows where to look for you. The pressure for an untrained bicyclist like me to keep up was tremendous.

I was interviewed by two TV stations – Channel 8 and Channel 12. I loved that part! Gabriel waited up until the 10:00 p.m. news to video the interviews. Yours truly was snoozing by then.

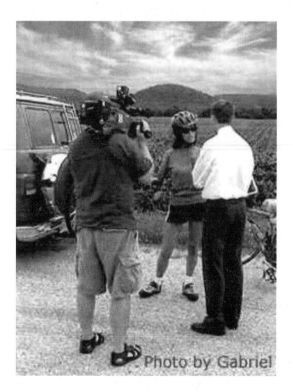

Photo by Gabriel

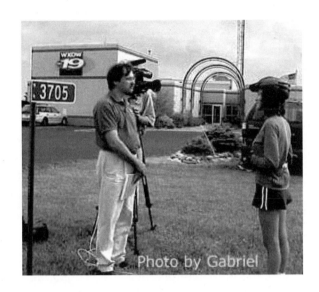

Before we got to LaCrosse, we crossed the Mississippi River for the first time. The bridge over the river was frightening. It was made of metal grates. I could see through the grates all the way down to the Mississippi below. Traffic whizzed by my left side. A solid concrete railing was on my right. I was terrified, but had to keep going as there was no place to stop. It definitely was not the same perspective you would have cruising across the bridge in a car. By the time I rode off into the new state, Wisconsin, my legs were shaking. They felt like tubes full of Jell-O. I understood why some of the cyclists refused to ride over bridges. They either walked or waited for the sag wagon. I'd try anything to enable me to pedal every inch of America.

I had now cycled through five states! Wow!

Day 33:
LaCrosse, WI to
Wisconsin Dells, WI

92 miles.

I needed a spare – and it wasn't a rubber tire. I'm referring to the saying we have nine lives.

I now had only eight.

While riding through Union Center, a small friendly city, I was intently watching a black SUV backing down a long driveway on my right. Usually a driver will come down quickly and then decelerate, pause and look before backing onto the street.

As I watched the car continuing at a fast pace, I tried to figure out what my maneuver was going to be. The vehicle was neither braking nor slowing. The drama compounded quickly as a semi truck rolled up beside me on my left and a concrete bridge abutment loomed in front of me. The black SUV continued to barrel down the long driveway.

The entire scene happened in a matter of seconds.

My natural instincts completely flip-flopped. I've been driving since age fifteen and have successfully maneuvered out of many scary situations to keep autos and drivers in one piece and unblemished.

My usual modus operandi was to hit the brakes and gain a few extra seconds to assess the situation before making a decision.

That day, however, as I realized I was about to become a sandwich in a place I didn't want to be in, my instincts went into gear. Instead of braking, I stepped on the gas – my pedal

154

power – and shot out of the situation with Lance Armstrong speed. I was instantly propelled out of there as if by rocket fuel. The big semi beside me became a blur; and I narrowly missed the concrete bridge abutment. I heard the horrible screeching of brakes behind me, as the semi and the black SUV started to deal with each other, but I didn't stop to see the conclusion. I wasn't the cause of the trouble, and also knew I had escaped by the "hair on my chinney-chin-chin."

Gabriel was several miles ahead of me on the other side of town. When I caught up to him, my normally pink cheeks were absolutely white. He asked, "Baby, what's wrong?"

I blurted out, "I almost got killed! I used up one of my nine lives." I told him my body had made an incredible decision on its own. I was scared, shaky, crying, and upset; it took him half an hour to get me calmed down and ready to get back on the road. I finally slipped back on my bike again after thanking my guardian angel for keeping me safe. I had many more miles to conquer and places to see. I pedaled on with a never to-be-forgotten panic tucked into my soul.

We never knew how each day would unfold. The first day of riding in Wisconsin consisted of terrain more rugged than Minnesota but still full of corn and soybeans. The weather was cool, unusual for midsummer in the Midwest. I was tired after pedaling four days of around a hundred miles each, and grateful I didn't have to cope with the heat.

As we rode through the Elroy-Sparta area (the Bicycling Capital of America), we saw such a unique drinking fountain.

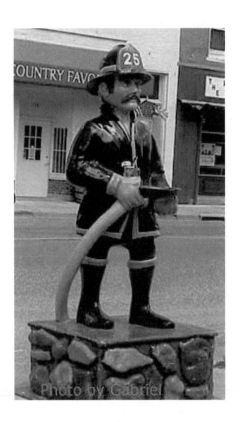

The day had started on a picturesque bicycle trail. The state of Wisconsin had a super idea when they utilized an abandoned railroad bed to build a spectacular bikeway meandering through the hills and valleys. What an admirable concept to use something that's already there for the enjoyment of so many others. Along with the scenario were three abandoned railroad tunnels. The longest was three-quarters of a mile. That tunnel, incredibly, was built by hand in 1872.

As we entered the tunnel, we had to walk and push our bicycles. A sign posted at the entrance stated that riding a bicycle was prohibited, as it was too dangerous. The proverbial light at the end of the tunnel was a pinpoint in the far, far distance. Blackness swallowed us. Not only was darkness a factor, but the track itself was raised in the center, rough, and pitted with water-filled potholes. The edges slipped away on the sides into troughs filled with water. Condensation on the inside of the tunnel dribbled off the ceiling and plopped on our helmets and bodies. Sounds reverberated eerily back and forth through the emptiness, until I couldn't figure out where they were coming from or who was talking.

I've ridden many miles alone but was thankful someone from the group was at the entrance to "hold" the bicyclists until there was a group of five or six of us to wend our way through the darkness together.

It took half an hour to pick and place each step until we finally saw the pinpoint of light getting large enough to let us walk out of the darkness.

Gabriel and his camera never got to capture any of the scariness or beauty of the trail, as the vehicles had to proceed to the next sag stop via ordinary roads.

The other two tunnels were somewhat shorter in length so we felt like pros when we entered them, and the darkness didn't seem quite as eternal. It was impossible to feel and see the blackness of the railroad tunnels unless you were walking by my side.

I certainly wouldn't want to be in there on Halloween night! Boo!

Day 34:
Wisconsin Dells, WI to
Fond du Lac, WI

84 miles

I spent the morning pedaling in the most idyllic setting of farmland. The first forty-four miles were a treat, except for pushing hard to climb those eternal long rollers as we got closer to the Great Lakes.

Innovative mailboxes were the fashion. Some looked like a fish, others like a baby tractor, or a car engine with hoses dangling out of it. The long, cold days of winter must spark imaginations.

There were many farm animals and huge barns of turkeys. Happy Thanksgiving to someone!

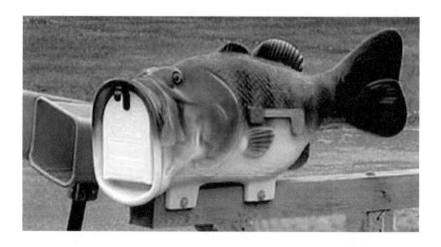

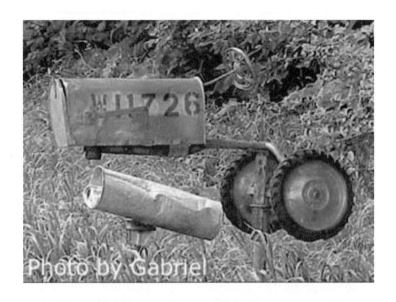

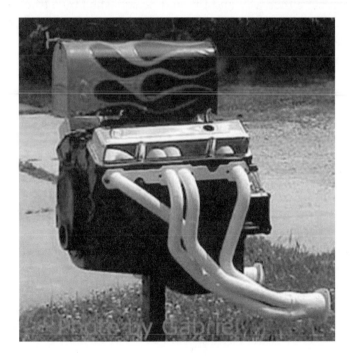

The afternoon was a test in concentration. I spent the last forty miles on CR-23, which means "country road." It sounded like a great afternoon as many of them have little traffic and it's possible to pedal and sightsee at the same time.

Did I get a surprise, and it wasn't a good one. CR-23 turned out to be a heavily trafficked road with many trucks hurtling past. The only place to ride was a strip on the right side of the white line that was only two feet wide. The edge of the pavement dropped down about six inches into really soft dirt and gravel. My mind knew exactly what would happen if I got mixed up with that combination. It would stop my bicycle and throw it on its side immediately.

There was no alternative but to keep my head down and concentrate for the next four hours. One little waver of my bicycle either way and I would be squashed by a truck or land face down in the dirt. I didn't see another thing all afternoon except the white line and the narrow strip leading to Fond du Lac, the next destination.

Day 35:
Fond du Lac, WI to
Manitowoc, WI

57 miles

There was hope! A reasonable day was on the agenda.
The other good news was a rest day at the next destination that
included a four-hour ferry ride across Lake Michigan. It's
amazing how I had changed my thinking. Riding the half-
century ride in Solvang, CA, a few years ago, was utter torture
and a huge accomplishment. Now fifty plus felt like a fluff day.

We had a luxurious 8:00 a.m. departure. The Ramada
Inn where we stayed was in the downtown area. It had been
completely refurbished to enhance its "old" look. There was a
gorgeous grand piano in the lobby to add to the elegance.
While waiting, I was eager to sit down and let my beautiful
Chopin music flow through the area. The experience will be
remembered instead as "heartbreak hotel." I knew my fingers
were feeling strangely stiff from curling around the handlebars
all of those days. I didn't know it was impossible to make them
move over the keys. My brain gave the same commands it
always did as I performed, but the fingers were like solid
blocks that refused to obey. I was stunned. What had I done to
myself?

Was my career as a performer over because of my crazy
whim to pedal America? As I held back my tears of frustration
and fled from the piano, I went to look for the doc who was the
kidney transplant surgeon. He was going back to work
immediately after the ride was over. Were his skilled fingers

161

feeling the same way? When I did find him, he noticed I was upset.

"Patricia, what's wrong?"

"Doc, I need to talk to you. When I tried to play the piano in the lobby, my hands wouldn't respond at all. It must be what people feel when they've had a stroke. I immediately thought of you. What about your hands?"

"Patricia, I was really bummed having to ride the sag for five days, but my hands are fine because of the enforced break."

My angel must have been looking out for him too, I thought.

"I understand your anxiety, but as an experienced cyclist, I can assure you, your hands will relax. You have to be patient with yourself. It probably will take a few weeks after you get off the ride."

All three docs were great – they had been an additional support to all of us "pedalers." Many others had assorted problems as we stressed our bodies to the max.

Detours again – every day was an adventure. It was never about turning the pedals around as I maneuvered from point A to point B. Finding myself again on the map was always a challenge. I arrived at 1:30 p.m. and had to wait two hours before our room was ready. Was that really me sitting on the leather couch in the lobby? I even beat Gabriel by a few hours. Did I ever feel smug!

The shortened day came at a perfect time. We actually went out to dinner in the evening with friends who lived in the area. It had been thirty-nine days since we'd had the opportunity to do so. The one objective, to cross America, was all consuming because of those long hours on the road. We had now conquered six states. Unbelievable!

Day 36:
Manitowoc, WI to
Ludington, MI

Rest day plus 7 miles

What fun - the wind blowing my hair and caressing my cheeks and I only needed to stand there to enjoy it. The ride across Lake Michigan was fabulous. The vast lake reminded me of the Pacific Ocean. The weather was perfect; our bicycles were tucked safely below deck; the ambiance made it a spectacular rest day.

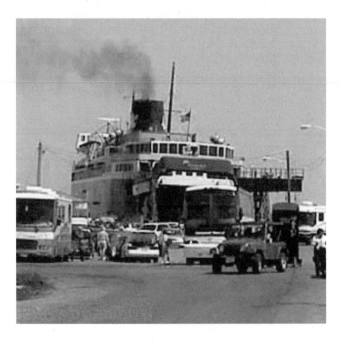

Gabriel and I spent the first couple of hours on the top deck enjoying the breeze. We strolled around the boat and stepped into the cafe to get some lunch. While we were eating, I noticed a table of all female cyclists from our group. Our days had been so long and focused on riding there had been no chance to gab.

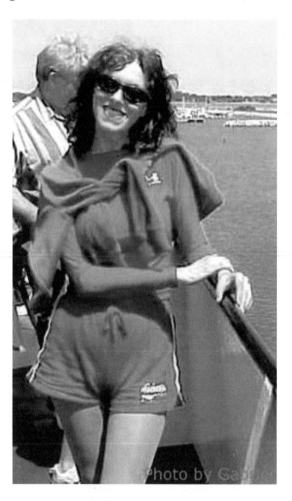

Gabriel walked out onto the deck, but one of the gals beckoned to me, "Come and join us."

When I sat down, Carolyn said, "Patricia, I've been dying to talk to you. I've heard you are married to a much younger man. I've read stories and seen talk shows about the subject, but never met anyone who has really done it. I'm sure you know the other bicyclists are curious too."

I responded, "I didn't go looking for a man 20 years my junior, it just happened. Gabriel was my mechanic, and every girl loves and depends on someone who can take good care of her car and not rip her off. The first time I saw him, I thought he was the handsomest, sexiest guy I'd ever seen. I'm a sucker for dark skinned guys with white smiles anyway. Then I discovered he was nice too! When he found out I was a musician and teacher, he started taking piano lessons from me. He had enjoyed music as a kid but let it go during his 'macho' years, although the love was still there. We became best friends because of our mechanic/teacher relationship but nothing further than that. He was newly married and so was I."

Melanie chimed in, "Is he as sexy as he looks?"

"He sure is. I don't know any woman who wouldn't love having great sex every day."

They all giggled. I continued, "Many years later, he told me when he was having a piano lesson, he wished he could put his hand on my leg; but knew he couldn't or shouldn't and didn't."

Jenny piped up, "But aren't you worried about what will happen when you get old – you know what I mean. I guess you already are, but you surely don't look or act like you're 67."

"Jenny, some of Gabriel's friends used to make snide remarks about 'the old lady in the wheel chair' that he was dating. Little did they know that old lady would be pedaling her butt across America."

Sandra asked, "What about your mother-in-law? I heard that you're older than she is!"

165

"You're right. I'm sure she thought her son was really crazy when she found out we were having a romance that was headed for matrimony. His family hadn't spoken to him for years, because they believed all the lies his former wife spread about him. They had plenty of time to get used to the idea."

I continued, "What matters is the relationship between the two people. Age doesn't need to be a part of it. None of us control the moment we enter this earth. We are who we are the moment we are born. I had never dreamed there was a possibility for us. I, like you, had only read about it in magazines. Both of our marriages had broken apart. I was always fascinated by him: his looks, the way he treats people with respect, his creativity and a mind that never stops. I didn't know that Gabriel had a supportive older female friend since his teenage years. He had no stigma about age as many guys would. The older man/younger woman concept seemed acceptable everywhere. Why shouldn't the flip side work as well?"

April asked, "What about your kids, Patricia?"

"I only have one son--he's six years younger than Gabriel, but has always been his own person, and thought it was cool as long as 'his Mom' was happy. Michael has fun calling my husband 'Pops', and they are both hands-on men with innovative minds that get along great." I checked my watch. "It's been fun talking with you," I said, "but it's time to go topside and find my boy-toy."

"Thanks, Patricia," they all chimed. "We were just curious."

Meanwhile, Gabriel had been telling a woman and her daughter about me; and when I appeared, they excitedly asked for my autograph.

We boarded in Wisconsin and landed in Michigan, ready to bicycle our seventh state! Disembarking was a slow process followed by a short seven mile ride to our hotel. The remainder of the day was spent mentally preparing for the long 115 miles to Mount Pleasant.

Day 37:
Ludington, MI to
Mount Pleasant, MI

115 miles

Rain, rain, and more rain. It was pouring – or as they say in mid-western vernacular – it was raining cats and dogs. As we ate breakfast, lightning streaked through the sky and thunder boomed down so hard it rattled our dishes. When we stepped outside the restaurant, our director wouldn't let us leave because of the electrical storm. After twenty minutes, the thunder was only a few low growls, but the rain continued relentlessly.

Several bicyclists pedaled out into the deluge, then a few more. By the time I got my courage up, only a few of us remained. After a few blocks, I was drenched – as wet as if I had dived into a swimming pool. Even my bra and panties were soaked and my socks were squishing in my shoes.

Are we having fun yet?

The eternal question for bicyclists is "How much do you cover up?" You get wet if you do and you get wet if you don't. Any plastic or vinyl material traps perspiration inside – if rain can't get in, moisture can't get out. Your clothes were completely sopped either way. One of the bicyclists had the right idea. He said he didn't worry about it – his body was waterproof. I thought about his comment every time it sprinkled.

The biggest concern in the rain was the slippery riding surface. We had to be super careful. We were looking forward to the last "over 100-mile day." It was an extremely long one, however, because of the weather conditions and an additional detour at the end of the day. Those extra miles never seemed to end.

The "rollers" were starting to shorten here in Michigan. That meant one hill to climb after another – they were continuous.

I was talking to a friend last night and he asked, "Did the miles on the boat yesterday count in your 3,622 total?"

I responded, "Absolutely not! We only added seven miles to the tally yesterday as we pedaled from the boat to our hotel in Ludington."

I was amazed to see more farm land than anything else. It was beautiful and clean and green but not as manicured as Minnesota and Wisconsin. I usually thought of Michigan as all "big city" i.e. Detroit. The opposite is true. As I pedaled along, there would be a 50 mile stretch without any stores or services. I wondered how the farmers managed to keep their vehicles fueled. Desolate Wyoming had many of those blank stretches, but I was surprised to see the void in Michigan.

Day 38:
Mount Pleasant, MI to
Birch Run, MI

75 Miles

This was a pleasant day also. The rain was gone and the sun was shining, but it was still cool. It was unbelievable to be riding on a mid-summer day with a windbreaker on. I do thank the "bicycle gods" for that. The heat we'd endured on many of the days was an overload to my system. Somehow, I had survived. The heat had been a concern back when I had started dreaming of pedaling America, but my desire overruled my fears.

My windbreaker had become an "item" as I always seemed to be the unconventional bicyclist. My mid-section has little fat so the wind cooled me extremely fast. With the zipper up, heat was trapped in my body and my clothes get soaked. With the zipper down, my tummy froze. Why not turn my wind breaker around so the front is closed to keep me warm, and the back is open to let out body heat? It worked perfectly; but it is impossible to buy apparel designed like that. Consequently, I wore my jacket like a kindergartener who didn't know any better. Many who rode up to me asked the same question, "Why is your jacket on backwards?' As I explained, most said, "That makes sense. Someone should design something that works."

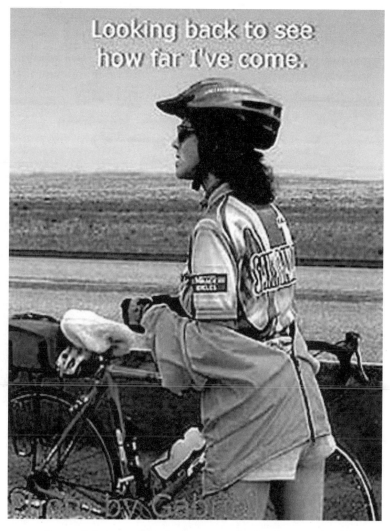

Looking back to see
how far I've come.

One of the women, however, who had owned a bicycle clothing shop said, "Patricia, that really looks stupid." I had a goal and planned to succeed even if I was a non-conformist!

I made it to the destination by 1:30 p.m. I even beat Gabriel again!

171

Late afternoon, I had a phone interview with the Saginaw News. Their reporter, Jeff Schrier, came out and took pictures of my bicycle and me by the van adorned with the stickers. The article and pictures should be in the paper tomorrow. My handsome PR man scored again!

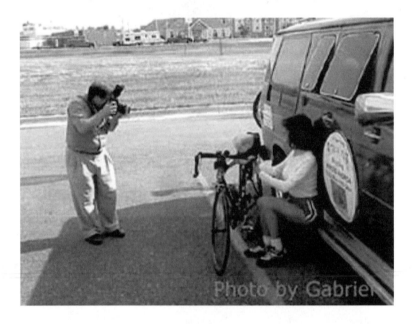

Ironically, that was to be the last printed picture of the beloved "Love Machine." Little did we know what was in store for us.

Day 39:
Birch Run, MI to
Port Huron, MI

89 miles

Thirty-nine days – the reality of what I had accomplished was overwhelming! I felt like Moses wandering in the wilderness for forty days! He was in the desert; I'd done that, too, but I'd also had other topographical challenges.

The day was almost another century and like the two previous days, miles and miles without any services. I rode sixty miles by noon. Other cyclists congratulated me for improving. Too bad I hadn't been that fit when I started in Astoria. Maybe I should go back and start over. Sheer determination and knowing I had the support of so many friends fueled my success. I was so grateful to still be on my bicycle and pedaling.

I pulled into Port Huron, the seventh state I'd conquered. Hooray!

Gabriel followed me and we were lost, as usual. When we stopped at a small shopping center to ask directions, the cutest sign caught our attention. It had the usual red and white striped barber pole on it, but the wording was "The Doggie Barber, Dog Grooming." A nice gentleman was standing nearby. I said, "I love your sign."

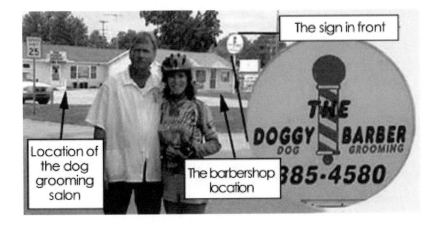

"Well," he replied, "There's nothing wrong with the sign, but it's the placement. That isn't my sign. It sits right in front of my business but I am a regular barber shop. I don't want that sign there because people can't find me. The landlord won't do anything about it. I've been frustrated about that sign for years." I guess everyone has their own problems!

We had a tiny glimpse of Lake Huron and the bridge that would take us into Canada. Some of the group, still freaked out by heights, will be in the center of the pack and try to forget where they are. It was exciting to think about riding in Canada for three days. The dream continues...

Day 40:
Port Huron, MI to
London, Ontario,
Canada

76 miles

What a thrill – the huge bridge from the United States to Canada was closed, so we bicyclists, for the first time, could ride over as a group without dodging traffic.

Surrounded by all the red, white, and blue jerseys with stars on them made my body tingle. I'd been resigned to my position as the caboose, but I had a chance to be like everyone else that morning.

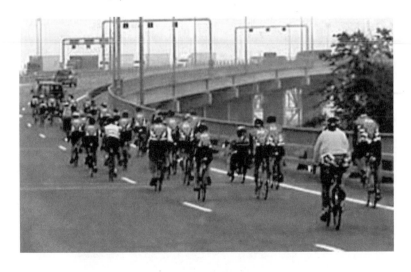

What a day – to start with, because our crossing time was at 8:15 a.m., we got to snooze a couple of extra hours. The four vans were with us. Even Gabriel was out early.

Everything went smoothly through customs, and we all experienced the grandeur of the huge structure of the bridge. A light drizzle had made the bridge extremely slippery. We had to be extra cautious.

As we started cycling in Canada, the farmland looked like America. The difference was the houses. They were either brown brick with beige trimming or beige brick with brown trimming. The bricks must only come in two colors.

There was an exception. Pedaling around a curve, I thought I was dreaming. There was a "California-looking" house with flowers everywhere. The mailbox was completely encircled with blooming orange impatiens. I'm a long-time gardener but had never seen the hanging plastic mesh bags filled with dirt so flowers can grow places other than in the ground or in pots.

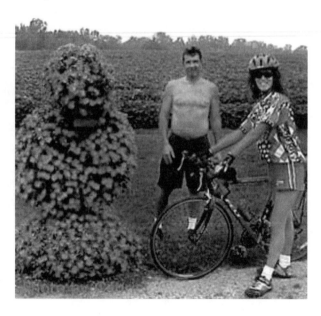

As I stopped to admire, the owner walked down the driveway, so we started to chat. Then Gabriel drove up and the farmer offered to show us around the property. His back yard had a Jacuzzi, ferns, flowers, meandering walkways and unbelievable color everywhere. The owner's wife joined us. They had a business on the property in a huge barn/warehouse structure where they designed and made artificial flowers for mailing all over the world.

They also promised to send me some of the plastic mesh bags, so I could grow hanging impatiens wherever I chose.

Where was I? It looked like California but my map said Canada.

Day 41:
London, Ontario to Brantford, Ontario

64 miles

I never realized Canada was a large tobacco grower. Fields rolled on forever. Sorry, bad pun! The rain and mist continued, but the coolness was ideal for pedaling. Bucolic was the perfect word to describe the day. How could I possibly envision the ruthlessness and heartache that soon was going to encompass us?

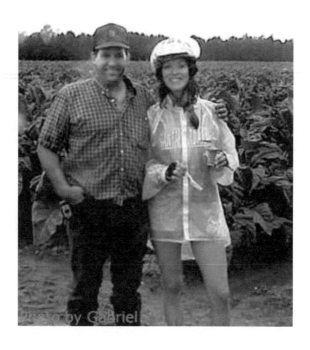

Day 42:
Brantford, Ontario to
Niagara Falls, NY

72 miles

Brantford, Ontario: A name and place never to be forgotten, the "un-highlight" of my Across America bicycle trip.

The sky had a faint glow, as I quietly started my morning routine. My shoes were sopping wet from riding in the rain the day before. About 6:10 a.m., I nudged Gabriel, "Would you pretty please get my dry shoes out of the van?"

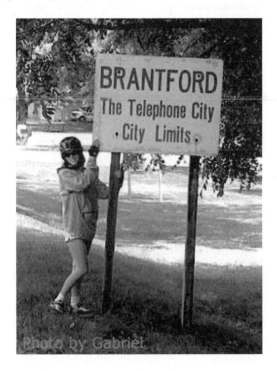

I scrambled around to get water bottles filled, rain gear folded, nuts to snack, gloves, glasses, and sunscreen while waiting for sleepy Gabriel to come back.

That morning he barged in the door yelling, "Baby, the van is gone."

I snapped, "Sure, knock it off. Don't be teasing me at 6:15 in the morning."

The look on his face told me something else – he wasn't teasing.

I tore off down the hall, minus my shoes, to the front desk. "Call someone! Our van is gone. It was parked twenty feet outside the door and it's not there." The sleepy, startled clerk probably thought I'd had too much tequila the night before. But he saw the tears running down my face and quickly realized something serious was happening. He asked, "Are you sure you remembered where you parked it?"

I sobbed, "Yes, twenty feet outside of our door."

By now Gabriel had caught up, and a few other bikers were gathering in the lobby. The clerk quickly dialed the constables. Word spread as more bikers appeared out of their rooms with their bikes.

Two Canadian cops were there in five minutes. The usual morning din and patter of happy bikers was gone. The silence, except for my sobs, was deafening. The constables got the usual details and kept asking, "Are you sure you know where you left it?"

Of course we were sure. We had been in the van about 9:00 p.m. the night before to get a snack. Then we locked it up for the night. As one of the constables was getting description information from Gabriel, his partner asked me to show him exactly where we had left it. We went outside.

When we got to the parking spot, I noticed a cook's helper smoking a cigarette outside the restaurant section of the building. He saw me crying and knew something was wrong, so he walked over. I sobbed, "Our van is gone. It was parked right there."

He said, "I saw a blue van with pictures on all four sides parked there when I came to work this morning at 5:30, and it was there when I came out at 6:00."

It was now about 6:20 so we knew the van had only been gone a short time. That made me feel a little better. No other van looked like ours. If they put out an APB, someone would recognize it.

Gabriel had been driving it for seven weeks since we left Santa Barbara to head north to Astoria, Oregon. He was so proud of the van. He had replaced everything on it except the motor to minimize any problems along the way. It had new carpet and paint, mag wheels, and those four big stick-on signs.

That was even the second set of signs. During some of the nasty storms we went through, the signs peeled apart, much to Gabriel's disgust. He had spent hundreds of dollars on them. After many calls back and forth with the company, they FedEx'd an entire new set to replace the ones that hadn't survived the rains.

The Love Machine was so dubbed by the guys at GM Automotive. It was an '86 van used, loved and well cared for by one of our customers. Colored light strips extended all the way back and across the ceiling. It looked like Christmas or Las Vegas.

The customer wanted a new one, and Gabriel knew everything about the van. We had owned it for five years and had many fond memories of and in it.

It was now 6:30 a.m., and the bikers had started to hit the road. We had been looking forward to riding over Rainbow Bridge into the City of Niagara Falls in the late afternoon, to enjoy one of the wonders of the world, and also to have a day off.

My stomach was tied in knots. My head throbbed from crying. Because of my hypoglycemia, I couldn't take off

181

without food, so I ran upstairs into the restaurant. The cyclists had left a few crumbs on the buffet table. I forced those crumbs down my throat. I knew I had to do what I knew I had to do – get on my bicycle and take off. So much had happened in those few minutes since I needed dry shoes that my head and body felt like they were spinning off into space.

I had to go on. I was pedaling for a music scholarship at Santa Barbara City College. The "Baron," the longtime DJ at 1290 AM, was sponsoring me on the radio station and keeping updates about my ride. Whenever I called him, he put me on the air "live."

John Palminteri at KEYT-3 was keeping Santa Barbarans informed with special spots. Charlotte Boeschler of the SB News Press had written a fabulous article the Sunday before we took off, and headlined me on the top of the front page beside Shaquille O'Neil and Tiger Woods. Barney Brantingham had included my saga in his daily column in the News Press. So many friends and family were rooting for me, even though at the beginning they all had thought I was crazy.

Could I call home and say I'm quitting?

I had ridden six weeks, 3,005 miles. Only 617 remained before the front bicycle tire could be dunked in the Atlantic Ocean. With a hug from Gabriel and his assurance that everything was going to be okay, I put on my helmet, wet shoes, gloves and glasses and took off with tears streaming down my cheeks. I was hoping my 45 SPF sunscreen was waterproof.

With everything happening so quickly, we didn't have time to absorb all the ramifications. The last ABB van was leaving Brantford in fifteen minutes.

What about my husband – we were not even in America – where could he buy wheels? And licensing? And cross the Canadian border by himself?

He had no choice but to climb in the last van that hit the road. He was one more piece of luggage. Everyone was nice, but there was no freedom. There was always some cyclist needing assistance with flat tires or mechanical problems, or giving up for the day. Too bad if Gabriel was hungry or had to go to the bathroom.

Why was our van the target? The two ABB vans with small logos were parked ten feet away – one red and one white (and with our blue one we looked so patriotic in the parking lot.) Ours was not the van to be "incognito."

What about me, the gal who was riding America alone (most of the time)? ***Now I was going to be alone***. How could I survive the afternoon hours with no one to wet down my clothes when the temperature was blistering; no one to bring me food and cold water? My body needed fuel as much as the vans did. How could I go on without it?

Gabriel and the beautiful blue Love Machine were my only tie to reality. Because I was always so slow, three-fourths of the cyclists were already at the next hotel relaxing around the pool.

What about trying to get to the hotel by myself? We arrived in a new town during end-of-the-day traffic, and had to fight our way through the city to get to the hotel on the outskirts. Gabriel would already be there in the ABB van. The person riding "sweep" (checking on the last person out for the day), would not find me if I was lost and not on their map.

I had no idea where we were or where we were going. I didn't want to make a wrong turn and add more miles to an already l-o-n-g day. It was difficult enough to find the way with Gabriel's help.

I wasn't used to rush-hour traffic. In the hills above Santa Barbara where I had done my meager amount of training, I might see one or two cars every five miles.

My mind was spinning as I rode down the highway on my bicycle "Starfire." I assumed Gabriel's was spinning, as he rode in the back seat of the sag wagon.

What if they don't find the van? Oh, but they surely would – there was no other van like it. Thoughts ran through our minds over and over. What about everything inside the van? We had been on the road for two and a half months. We had brought our lives with us. Gabriel had packed every tool possible to make sure we had everything we needed. Being in the auto repair business, he knew the stories of people stranded in God-forsaken places in America. He had helped numerous motorists on the freeways and highways, while he was on the road waiting for me. He was the ultimate Good Samaritan.

And what about clothes? Now Gabriel only had the clothes on his back. As Gabriel had loaded and unloaded the van by himself, I had suggested, "Why do you lug your big suitcase in every night? Take out only the shirt and shorts you're going to wear the next day!" It worked for forty-one days, until that last night.

What about my clothes? I had my suitcase in the room with my bicycle stuff in it. My other clothes were another story.

In 1977, while I was away on vacation, a horrific California wildfire had burned down my house and everything in it. After that, every time I left for an extended time, I put my favorite clothes and accompanying jewelry in one suitcase in case my house disappeared in another inferno. Another bag held the matching shoes. After surviving a wildfire and losing everything in my possession, the scars were there of the trauma of having my life disappear – everything except what was in my head.

With the missing van, the scars were reappearing. My brain was spinning and my body and soul ached. How could I concentrate riding down a highway with traffic whizzing by my tush.

Gabriel's beautiful shiny new bicycle was locked on our new bicycle rack on the back of the van. We cyclists

184

always kept our bikes in our rooms. The umbilical cord wouldn't have reached out to the van.

What about the $2500 in cool cash hidden inside the air conditioning vent? We would never have to worry about anyone finding that if someone broke into the van.

We had packed our special books, records, pictures, DVD's, address books, cameras and equipment – I had to quit thinking and concentrate on getting to Rainbow Bridge, clearing customs and riding into Niagara Falls.

Since the beginning of the planning stages, that day was to be one of the highlights. Gabriel loved waterfalls. What could be more spectacular than Niagara Falls? I had seen it once on a college choir tour in early spring, when everything was barren and still frozen. It was the ultimate place for lovers. We were looking forward to enjoying the day together. Before we parted that morning, we both agreed no matter what happened during the day, we would not let it interfere with our dream day in Niagara Falls.

The cyclists felt my agony. Someone always made sure I was not riding alone.

As the day went on, one o'clock, two o'clock – I would hear a familiar engine coming up behind me; but then it would be someone else's Chevy van that would drive on by.

Somehow, I was able to keep riding. Thank God the weather was reasonable so I didn't need to be sprayed down. The knots in my stomach kept me from feeling any kind of hunger. The adrenalin in my body kept my blood sugar from plummeting as it normally would after so many miles on the road.

Many kept asking, "What enabled you to keep going, not only that day, but all of those challenging days? Are you for real?"

I think being a "cornhusker" and living the life of a farm family had something to do with it. After my father's sudden death at age 51, life was a real struggle for my mother and me; but we knew we had to go on alone.

I was so determined to ride across America that no matter what happened, I was going for it. Only being road kill myself would have stopped me.

Crossing the border on Rainbow Bridge was not a problem. Returning to America was a thrill, but as I tried to find my way to the hotel on the American side, I was inches from cars, going down a hill so steep I could hardly stand on it. Then the wonderful sounds I had been hearing came into view, and I saw one of the wonders of the world – Niagara Falls.

Our rooms were only a few short blocks from the Falls. When I got to the hotel and found Gabriel, we went out to see everything we could.

After dinner that night, we walked down to the Falls to see what they looked like with the night-lights on them. There were times in the midst of the beauty, we actually forgot about the trauma for a few moments.

We tried to console ourselves that we were safe. If the thieves were so brazen to steal in the daytime from a Holiday Inn, they probably had guns and didn't care about human life.

Memories of a few days ago when I was almost a sandwich between a car, a semi and a concrete bridge abutment made us even more aware of the important things in life.

We strolled through the arcade between the Falls and the room. I was ready to collapse from the drama and the ride of the day. I went back to the room alone. I took a leisurely bath and tried to quiet my mind about the fate of the van.

About 10:15 p.m. the phone rang. I raced to get it – almost too scared to answer. Who would call after 10 p.m? It was a constable on the phone.

She asked, "Are you both in the room?"

"No," I replied.

She responded, "I'll call back later."

186

I pleaded, "Will you please talk to me now? I know what this is all about."

She finally agreed and said, "They found the van about 6:00 p.m., twelve hours after it was taken."

My heart was flip-flopping so fast, I thought it was going to jump right out of my chest. The next sentence I heard was, "But it has been torched."

My world crashed. I couldn't believe what I was hearing. How could anybody destroy like that? I know people steal things all the time, but to steal and destroy is incomprehensible to me. I asked, "How can this happen?"

She responded, "It happens all the time."

I hung up the phone and sat there sobbing in a state of complete numbing shock. Gabriel didn't return for another half-hour; and when he opened the door and saw me, he didn't have to ask the fate of our beloved Love Machine.

At least we knew – otherwise we would have been looking at every blue van on the road, wondering if it was ours.

My pillow that night was as wet as my shoes were in the morning. All night long I kept waking and sobbing. I had my own Niagara Falls.

Day 43:
Rest Day at
Niagara Falls

BRIINNG! BRINNG! BRINNG! The shrill piercing
clang of a fire alarm resonated through the hotel. A knock on
our door and a hurried "Everyone evacuate the building
immediately" was heard through the closed door of our room.

Gabriel and I looked at each other in disbelief. That
couldn't really be happening. Only minutes before, we had
welcomed a reporter into our room. She was from the *Niagara
Falls Gazette*. She wanted the story about the stolen and
torched van.

We grabbed the few belongings we now had. The
reporter gathered up her equipment. We ran out into the hall
and down the fire escape as the alarms kept screeching.

As we waited outside, some of the cyclists were in the
group around us. Many tearful condolence hugs were shared as
the news had spread quickly that morning about our late night
phone call. No one could understand why something like that
had happened to us.

I was trying so hard to keep it together that morning.
After the tragic news, I hardly slept at all. How much more
could I endure? All my energy was being expended to survive
the physical challenges of each day. I didn't have any extra to
cope with the mental anguish that had suddenly befallen me.
Thankfully, I was healthy; but having to deal with the van loss
was scary. I knew I couldn't fall apart with only a week to go.
Losing the van and my afternoon support system was a
whopper.

After fifteen minutes of waiting and wondering what
was going on, a fireman came out of the building and told us

we could all return to our rooms. No one seemed to know what the scare was about, but we were relieved. Our shaken psyches didn't need any more traumas.

When we got back to our room, we all unloaded our arms and sat down to talk so the reporter could get the information she needed. She was shaking her head in disbelief. She was there to do a story about a torched van and got abruptly forced out of the building by a fire alarm.

Later that morning, we also had an interview outside our hotel with Channel 2.

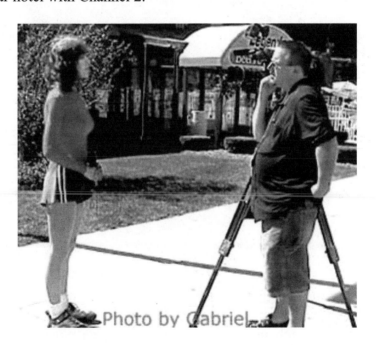

Photo by Gabriel

After the interview, we went back to the Falls. We wanted to get "into" the splendor as much as possible. We bought tickets and boarded the "Maid of the Mist," the boat that goes in back of the cascading falls. Everyone got a plastic raincoat for protection, as the mist was not only misty, it was wet. The sounds of the falling water and the enormous power as it fell were awesome. I felt like I was a part of the phenomenon.

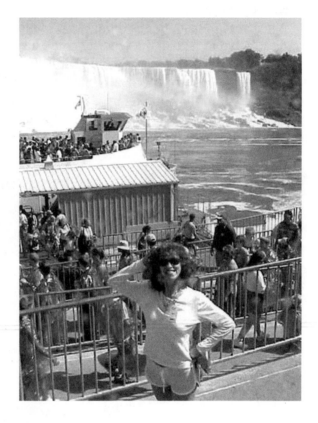

Hundreds of people were lined up behind ropes waiting for the previous passengers to disembark. When the signal came to climb aboard, everyone tried to get a spot at the railing. Gabriel and I found ours and were enjoying every second. The power, the roar of the water, and the brilliant colors as the water sparkled in the sunshine were an experience to remember forever.

I happened to turn around to look behind me and saw an older gentleman sitting all by himself on a bench in the center of the boat.

I told Gabriel, "Save my spot."

I wormed my way back through the crowd standing behind me, grabbed the old man's hand and led him back up to my place by the railing. He came willingly. We spent the entire ride huddled together under our plastics and helping each other keep our balance on the slippery deck. We had the best time and Gabriel got a great picture of us together. Wish I had his address; I would have sent him a picture.

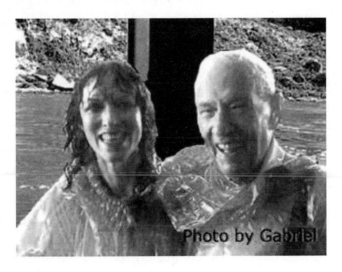

Photo by Gabriel

We had a nice dinner at one of the sidewalk cafes and absorbed every bit of Niagara Falls that we could. The day was full of tears but happy times also. We needed to let the rushing sounds of the water help soothe our battered souls.

We were grieving, but we had each other.

Day 44:
Niagara Falls, NY to Henrietta, NY

80 miles

My body ached from the turmoil. My heart was broken over the loss of my lifeline. My soul cried for the ugliness of the entire episode. Getting back on "Starfire," my bicycle, was the best therapy I could have had. There was nothing I could do about the theft, destruction and loss. I coped by letting the soothing hum of the tires, the softly falling rain, and my eternal spirit survive to carry me through the day. I had to find the physical, mental and emotional strength to go on.

How could anybody be so cruel and heartless as to steal and torch someone else's possessions? The first day back on the road after our Niagara Falls rest day was a blur of tears and sadness.

We had no idea who did it or why; but surely there would be karma for that someone - somewhere - sometime.

Gabriel finally got to talk to the towing company. They confirmed the van was completely torched and nothing remained inside. The fire was so hot the windshield had melted onto the engine.

The constables in Canada were absolutely no help when we tried to get information. We assumed they took pictures of our Love Machine for their files; but, when we asked for a picture, they said, "We didn't take any."

We had hoped there might be some belongings left in the van if and when it would be found. The fire took care of that. I'm sure no one found the $2500 in cash stashed "safely"

192

in the air conditioning duct. What an irony. That little discovery could have made their theft really worthwhile.

Now, the realization hit me hard: there *was* no one special on the road looking out for me. Even though on all the other days I hadn't seen Gabriel and the Love Machine for the first six or eight hours I was on the road, I knew he would be coming along. I'd listen for the familiar purring of the engine. It was the eternal hope I held on to no matter how distraught I was.

After the many hardships I've encountered and overcome in my life – my father's sudden death when I was eleven, being poor, surviving several divorces, losing all my belongings at age forty in a devastating fire – am I tough now? I knew I was not a quitter. That one thought got me back on my bicycle. I'd pedaled over 3,000 miles, a miraculous feat in itself, but nothing like the words "I pedaled America."

We are constantly reminded how small the world is. When I started writing this book, I enrolled in a writing class under our Adult Education system in Santa Barbara. I read the chapter about the van being stolen to the class.

The next week, a nice gentleman came up to me during the class break and commented on the chapter I had read the week before. He lamented about what a horrible thing it was to have had to endure. His next statement really shocked me.

He said, "Patricia, I know what happened to your van."

My mouth dropped.

I said, "How could you possibly know anything about my adventures while sitting here in a writing class in Santa Barbara?"

He countered, "I am in Santa Barbara for a few months to escape the cold weather in Canada. I live outside of Brantford where the van had been stolen at the Holiday Inn."

He continued, "There is an Indian Reservation about thirty miles from town. In the past, people had come into town from the reservation, stolen vehicles and driven them back on to the reservation and set fire to them"

I was in a complete state of shock. It was now over a year later and one of my classmates knew the answer no one was willing to tell us at the time of the theft. He clarified the reservation has its own governing system that differs from the Canadian system. They live side by side and ignore each other. That is the answer to *why* we could not get any information.

It also explained the cover-up the town was perpetrating. When we pedaled into Brantford several days ago, we noticed many boarded-up businesses indicating a "town in trouble." However, the AAA Holiday Inn appeased our fears as it looked respectable. No one told us a vehicle had been stolen the night previous to our stay even though Gabriel had asked the clerk, "Is my van safe in the parking lot?"

"Yes sir, of course," he replied.

If Gabriel had known the truth, he would have disabled the van so it couldn't be driven even if the lock system was by-passed.

The next week at writing class, another of my classmates handed me a photo of a burned out hulk. Oops, there came some more tears. He had heard last week's conversation between the Canadian snowbird and myself when I said that I really had wished for a picture of the van for closure purposes and also to include in my book. The photo wasn't the Love Machine but it accentuated the stark reality that there was nothing left.

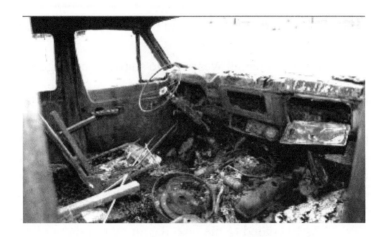

Last night, when I woke up sobbing at 2:00 a.m., my mind was randomly remembering the treasures tucked in my big suitcase in the van that no longer existed.

That suitcase was packed over seven weeks ago. I can't imagine what they did with my beautiful party clothes and performance gowns, and the sexy three-inch heels my husband loved. How long would it take me to find replacements for those items I'd collected over the years?

I had no intention of wearing the clothes on the tour; I knew we would always be "bicycle casual." The only reason they were with us was to keep them safe from a fire – how ironic!

The time lapse had made my inner vision of the suitcase kind of "fuzzy." So much had happened in those six weeks on the road, and none of it had been focused on what was inside of the suitcase.

My memory zeroed in on the beautiful blue shawl my mother and father-in-law had brought me from Barcelona, when they were in Europe the previous summer. It not only had sentimental value, it was gorgeous. The shade of blue looked like the Mediterranean Ocean on a bright, sunny day. It was

195

soft and silky with crocheted and braided fringe around the edges.

I felt so elegant wearing the shawl. It belonged in the "favorites" suitcase.

The saddest memory of all was the missing little red address book that my Mom had sent me after my home burned to the ground. She knew I had lost contact with everyone, so she wrote all the family names and addresses in a new book. It was my link to the past. Now, it, too, was gone.

I had to talk to myself all day: "Patricia, stop crying. You have something important to do – staying alive."

As I pedaled to the next destination, I did a pretty good job of holding back tears at least so I could see. Nothing could help the heavy heart that was beating under my bicycle jersey.

There was always some sunshine in the day. I especially remember the love and care of my fellow bicyclists. They took turns again making sure I didn't ride alone. They were holding back to match my slower pace.

They knew I was still fragile. The van disappearance was a numbing shock for everyone.

I had to force myself to eat to keep up my pedal strength, not an easy task with a stomach churning from the emotional turmoil and a stuffed-up head from crying. I surely wasn't feeling in top shape – either emotionally or physically.

Because concentration is the one essential a cyclist must have on the road, the day was a struggle from beginning to end.

When I had ridden two days ago from Brantford to Niagara Falls, I was lucky I made it without incident. We still had hope someone would find the van and we would get it back, maybe minus a few stripped items.

Now, hope had vanished and the reality was settling in. I still had my dream to pedal across America – _no one could steal that_. I had to keep my cool to finish those last 465 miles.

That added to the list of challenges I had faced since the first pedal out of Astoria, Oregon. I also knew I had to do the rest of the trek without Gabriel's assurance. He would be trapped in the sag wagon somewhere along the seemingly endless road.

When I pedaled into the hotel parking lot in Henrietta, New York, I really came unglued.

No matter how many times my eyes scanned the parking lot, the Love Machine was not there. When I had ridden to Niagara Falls the day the van was taken, our hotel was on the waterfront so I pedaled up to the front door. Now the barren parking lot had to be faced for the first time.

The beloved Love Machine, my lifeline, no longer existed.

It was not a bad dream – it was reality.

I was inconsolable.

Day 45:
Henrietta, NY to
Syracuse, NY

83 miles

Talk about timing and my guardian angel. I was usually by myself in the middle of nowhere. I had spent hundreds of hours alone during the past six weeks. However, my angel was there when I was in serious trouble. I started crying out, "Please, please, someone help me."

Another cyclist had crossed the bridge half a minute before me, and had stopped on the other end to get a drink. She heard me crying for help and raced back. She got on the phone immediately to call the sag wagon at the same time yelling, "Biker down."

That biker was me.

I lay there, not knowing if my world had come to an end. Had I ripped off my breast? Had I broken my leg? I assumed my head was OK, because I was conscious. I knew I was alert, as I felt more pain than I had ever experienced in my life.

How the distance of one-inch can change your world so quickly.

Last night had been another night of fitful sleeping. I was still upset about our van. Little did I know I was about to suffer an extreme physical problem to deal with on the road.

That morning was one of those treats a bicycle rider fantasizes about – a twenty-five mile bikeway along the Erie Canal. I remember singing the folk song about the "Erie Canal"

198

when I was in the one-room country school in Nebraska. Who would have dreamed I would be cycling there one day.

The entire area looked like it did in pictures: mottled stonework, old concrete, Mother Nature's luscious landscape and water that reflected like a mirror. I felt as though beauty surrounded me on all sides.

There were homes along the bike path that looked like they had been there forever. Their yards flowed gracefully from the property to the bike path and on down to the canal.

People walked along the pathway and stopped to talk. They had seen many bikers, but I was the one who stopped to chat to find out what could be gleaned from the locals.

I learned the canal was drained every fall except for a foot of water; otherwise, when the temperature dropped below freezing, the ice would crack the locks. The canal had been built for commercial purposes, but now was used for pleasure boats only. Plans to develop an inland waterway to link the Great Lakes to the Atlantic Ocean were developed in 1783, but progress was stalled until New York State agreed to fund the project. The first successful run from Lake Erie to New York City arrived in November of 1825.

Even though the bikeway was slippery gravel, to be able to ride along and not have to think about traffic for a few hours was heavenly. The pungent smells of the lush overgrowth wafted through the air. With the recent rains, it was a paradise.

I approached the end of the bikeway; it ended at a T intersection. The bushes and trees obscured any sort of vision to the right, making it a blind turn.

As I turned right, there was a concrete bridge for cars to transverse the canal and a pedestrian walkway to share the bridge. Between the two was the usual metal guardrail with the smooth side facing the cars, and the backside with naked bars facing the walkway.

I still wasn't functioning 100 percent. Some of those pesky tears were creeping out. It added up to pilot error of one inch that forced my bike tire to catch the edge of the bridge railing. In a second, it stopped both my bike and me.

My body flew forward and my left breast slammed into a sharp metal stanchion. As the pain seared through my body, I guess I felt the pain the male gender feels when kicked in their private parts. It was incredibly debilitating.

The next few seconds threw my body and bike into the next set of support poles and a few more slaps into the railing as body and bike tumbled again. We were so entwined, I was trapped and couldn't move.

My bike bent out of shape from the impact and smashed the handlebars into my left thigh. My legs were bruised and bleeding and my mind was screaming in pain with the thought my breast had been ripped off.

Word spread quickly, both forward and backward; there was "a biker down." Over the next few minutes, a crowd started gathering around me. The sag was twenty minutes ahead, but stayed on the phone with the caller while they turned around to come back.

Nobody moved either my bike or me immediately, as no one knew what kind of condition I was in. They knew I was in serious trouble and in a lot of pain. My friend Judith was trying to comfort me.

Then my angel worked another miracle.

There were two "docs" in the group of riders. Actually there were three, but one had returned to work for two weeks and would join again to finish the last few days. They had been in medical school together over twenty years ago and had reunited to pedal America.

One was a kidney transplant surgeon from the San Francisco area, another was an emergency room physician in downtown Detroit, and the third was an anesthesiologist. He was the one who had left the tour temporarily.

These guys were all in great shape and excellent bikers. I saw them at breakfast, when they waved to me as they pedaled by me, and again at dinner. The only day contact we had was the friendly wave.

That day was the exceptional day. They had decided to take a side trip in the morning. A few minutes after I went down, guess who came riding up from behind!

They immediately took over; got me off the walkway, sat me down and went to work. Each one took a side and patted me down from top to bottom, every muscle, bone and joint. No broken bones.

After they got down to my toes they said, "Okay, Patricia, look down into your shirt."

I was petrified to peek. They didn't want to look with a bunch of cyclists standing around, not quite the usual medical set-up. I didn't even have a gown on that opened in the back. My clothes looked okay except for my ripped Hanes support hose.

I remember swallowing really hard, pulling my shirt out at the neck, and peering down inside. I was expecting a bloody mess. Miraculously, I still had two breasts and there was no blood. The horrible pain was inside my body and that would heal. I knew at that moment I would not stop trying for my dream to pedal America.

The docs cut my Hanes hosiery so they could bandage the "owies" on my legs and then made me sit there for half an hour. I remember feeling extremely "dazed." The pain racing through my body was incredible.

How could I have been so lucky, not only to have all my parts still attached, but also to have the wonderful doctors there when I really needed help – my own Mayo Clinic on wheels.

The only one that couldn't be there was Gabriel. He was in the front sag wagon and heard about the crash over the two-way radio, but had no wheels to come back to me.

201

He later told me he had goose bumps over his entire body and had tears running out of his eyes when he heard the biker was Patricia. The sag he was riding in was going the other direction to help someone else. He had always been there for me with the Love Machine.

Now he was helpless.

Gabriel was the only person who had seen and experienced my struggles of pedaling across America. He knew how hard I had worked to pedal up all those hills and mountains—surviving the traffic, big trucks, lightning, hail, rain and heat.

He was watching when a terrific wind blew my bicycle and me over as I was riding over the long, scary bridge into Casper, Wyoming. Now, was the whole dream of pedaling across America, every inch, going to be aborted by a crash? With only five days to go?

The closest sag had turned around to come back. Mike, the director, was driving that one. He was always concerned when one of his chickens went down. After he knew the docs were taking care of me, he started working on my bicycle to get it straightened out, and the gears and chains repaired. A complete bicycle repair shop in his van enabled him to work his miracles.

While all that was happening, the other cyclists stayed around. We were like a pack of animals: if someone was in trouble, everyone was there. That would not have been the usual scenario. They were usually way ahead of me, while I was riding in the back of the pack by myself, the slow but steady diesel.

When the situation seemed to be under control, the other riders started moving on. It was an eighty-three mile day so there were many miles to go. A couple of cyclists stayed back with me.

As I sat there musing about what a difference an inch makes, my mind was flipping everywhere. I was so thankful to

202

be alive, to have no broken bones and two breasts. Now, after a serious accident, we would see about my true grit. It was up to me to handle it, no matter how much it hurt. I knew I was not a quitter.

It seemed like the theft and destruction of the van was the biggest calamity that could happen, but the crash disproved that.

One of the bikers had to go home two days earlier because of a broken arm. He had rammed the biker ahead of him while they were drafting (riding directly behind each other to lower wind resistance and increase speed). He did the natural thing when you go over, put your arm down to break the fall.

I was missing my real angel, Gabriel. He was now at the next rest stop, which was thirty miles down the road. He was going to be pacing back and forth for at least two and a half hours, maybe more, and could do nothing except wait and worry. He said he felt like a "Daddy" in the waiting room.

My half hour of imposed rest was up.

As I gingerly stood up, I knew my body wasn't the same body that had cruised effortlessly alongside the Erie Canal an hour ago. The only thing to do was get on my bike and start pedaling. I absolutely refused to get in the sag wagon with Mike. They say, "Swedes are stubborn." My heritage was showing.

The cuts and bruises were manageable. The pain in my breast was agonizing, but at least it wasn't being aggravated by motion. That left leg was another story. The constant, throbbing pain flooded my body, and every move intensified it.

I had to keep going. If I stopped, it was all over. Somehow, one pedal after another slowly propelled me to the next rest stop. At least Gabriel would be waiting there – I needed his strength. The only thing that made him smile was the thought that I was so determined to succeed; he knew I wouldn't be in the sag wagon unless I was dead.

The nagging thought I couldn't get rid of concerned the doc from San Francisco and his injury. Even all the docs at the Mayo Clinic couldn't keep him out of the sag. The leg had to heal on its own time, and that was five days.

Was that what was coming next for me? That would have meant the ride was over. I should have been icing my leg and keeping it elevated, but I only had 400 plus miles to go. Could I, should I, do the reasonable thing? Could it be expected of me? A 67-year-old broad with no experience pedaling across America – in itself, that was not reasonable.

When I pedaled into the parking area at the next sag stop, I couldn't get off my bike, because the injured leg wouldn't bend. It hurt so much that I couldn't stand on it to get off the other side either. I had pedaled the entire distance with my right leg. Luckily, there hadn't been any big climbs. Gabriel had to lift me off my bike. The director of physical medicine watched us. It was her job to see that riders were using good judgment and taking the best possible care of themselves.

When she saw me, she insisted I get in the sag wagon for at least the rest of the day, and then make a judgment about the remaining five days. How could I do that after I had worked so hard and long to pedal every inch of America?

We argued for a while. She realized I was not going to give in. I felt like a dog with all four paws firmly planted on the ground, refusing to get in the paddy wagon.

She said, "I don't agree with your decision. I have given you my medical opinion. I release my responsibility concerning the situation."

I said, "I understand your point and thank you for caring, but I have to keep trying. I will not quit now."

The sag wagon had to go on ahead and Gabriel had to go with it. There I was again, pedaling America alone. The rest of the day was a blur of pain. Somehow, the right leg got me to the next hotel in Syracuse, New York.

I was still unprepared to roll into the barren parking lot and not see the Love Machine. That truly had been my umbilical cord. Why couldn't I keep those darn tears away?

I limped into our room and collapsed on the bed. Gabriel brought me dinner in a doggie box. The restaurant was only a few blocks away, but it was impossible for me to walk. If the directors had seen how hurt I was, they would have pulled me off the ride. They always had the final word.

I remembered pedaling over the Continental Divide and the exhilaration after climbing to 9,683 feet. After that, I felt I could survive anything. Now I had to prove it.

I borrowed some ice packs to anesthetize my aching body. I rejoiced that I still had two breasts and two legs; and decided I'd deal with tomorrow, tomorrow!

Day 46:
Syracuse, NY to
Little Falls, NY

86 miles

"Tomorrow" had arrived. As I struggled out of bed, I had no idea how my body was going to make it through the day.

The pain in my throbbing leg was horrible. I had to ease onto my bike and take off. Once the leg started going around, the pain subsided a bit. I couldn't walk on it and stairs were impossible.

It's incredible how I survived so many days and then did something as stupid as hitting a railing.

I was thankful that I hadn't caused anyone else to crash or be injured.

Day 47:
Little Falls, NY to Troy, NY

70 miles

My leg had a little more flexibility, but I still couldn't walk correctly. I needed to stay close to someone so the leaders couldn't see how badly I was injured.

I had a little more excitement in the morning, a flat tire. Lucky for me, my friend Dan rode with me, and he changed the tire. There were actually other cyclists behind us. They were gathered around asking and laughing "is it dead yet?"

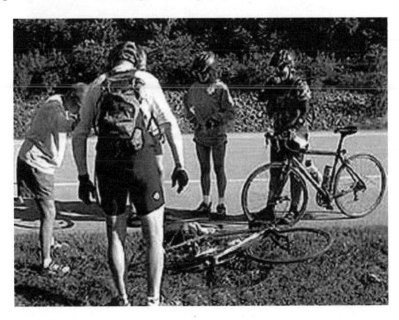

Riding that day was like being in fairyland. We were on a twenty-five mile bike path that was ethereal. The color and lushness of the foliage looked like a Technicolor picture with the rider in the middle. I felt like I was riding in green lace with the trees forming canopies over my head.

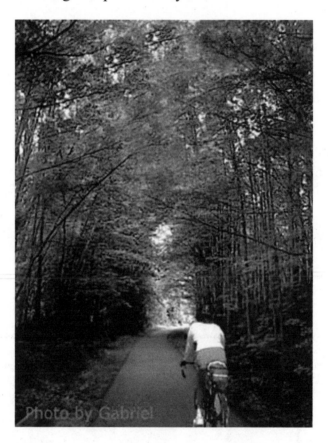

Mentally, the week had taken its toll. I almost hit another railing. As we crossed over the bridge, the netting on the side didn't sit on a two-by-four. It went down to the bridge floor itself. When I looked down, my eyes saw right through the mesh so it looked like there wasn't anything on the edge of the bridge. Instinctively, I moved away to the left and stopped just before hitting the rail. My crash two days ago had really shaken me. I needed time to get my confidence back.

We had an after dinner "Route Rap." Mike said we would not "coast to the coast." We had two serious days of climbing ahead. He reminded us that we had made it up Teton Pass and Togwotee Pass and we should be stronger after all those miles.

That was all true, but I wasn't hurting then.

I would not give up.

DAY 48:
TROY, NY TO
BRATTLEBORO, VT

81 MILES

Gabriel was acting like a puffed up rooster cock. He chided me, "I'll take it easy on you, Baby. If you can't keep up, I'll pull over and wait for you."

I said nothing.

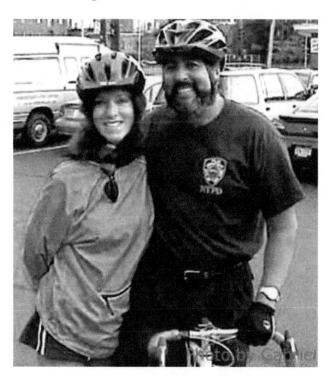

Fast forward to five o'clock.

Should I laugh or cry? The most handsome man I'd ever known was sprawled across the bed as I stumbled into our hotel room in time to get ready for dinner. He looked like a piece of road kill, and I'd seen plenty after keeping my head down and focused on the roadways for those many weeks.

The irony of the situation made me giggle, but the pain written all over his face and body made my heart ache. He barely mumbled as I hurried to the bed.

"Baby, are you OK?" I whispered. "I've been worrying about you all afternoon. I didn't know if you were passed out in a ditch somewhere or in the emergency room at the local hospital. Please talk to me."

Only a few faint sounds slipped from his lips. I didn't know if I should call 911 or watch over him myself as he lay there moaning.

That was the boy-teenager-man who had spent countless hours of his life on bicycles and motorcycles. Two wheels were not something new. The problem was, his mind hadn't comprehended what I and the other cyclists had been dealing with every day of our odyssey.

Gabriel only thought he knew what it felt like, as he pressed his foot on the gas pedal of the Love Machine. We cyclists could have filled him in on some of the details, but he never asked. Now he had a chance to feel what it really was like to be out there on the road all day.

But, wait, that last phrase needs to be clarified. He didn't make the entire day. He sagged into the hotel after mile fifty, less than half the distance we had pedaled on many days. What was that going to do to his manly pride when he finally emerged from his current torture?

Gabriel was getting fed up of being a piece of luggage in the ABB sag wagon. That had been his only option after our Love Machine was so ruthlessly stolen and burned in Canada five days ago.

211

ABB did carry an extra bicycle with them in case of emergencies. However, a new cyclist had joined us in Niagara Falls. When her bike came out of its shipping box to be assembled, a piece was missing. She needed the extra bike.

Gabriel was impatiently waiting for the day when the missing part would catch up with us so he could taste the "freedom" of taking off on a bike. As the days ticked off, so did the flat and gently rolling hills of middle and eastern New York State.

The other cyclists were trying to help in every way they could. They knew Gabriel had nothing to wear except the clothes on his back. Items kept appearing outside our door at night: a helmet, a pair of bicycle shoes with clip-on cleats, a pair of socks, bicycling gloves and a water bottle, the essential things needed for his "big ride."

Word finally came that the part had arrived. Gabriel would have his chance to be sprung from his cage. He easily made friends wherever he went, so he was already a popular member of the group. The cyclists were jiving with him and encouraging him to go for it. They knew he would be in for a rude awakening, but they were still behind him. Everyone felt badly for him, because he had ended up being "the third wheel." He had not only lost his van and possessions, he had lost his niche in the group itself.

He donned all the necessary gear that morning and looked and felt like one of us for the first time. He was smiling and happy and even went down to eat a little breakfast (not his usual routine).

I prudently said nothing about the day except that it would be fun to have him on the road with me. I loved being with Gabriel, and was so happy he had agreed to come along for the entire saga across America. I really didn't mind that he wasn't on two wheels.

He had been very adamant from the beginning that he didn't want to spend fifty days with that skinny bicycle seat stuck up his butt.

Everything was right about Gabriel's debut except the timing. We now had only three days left to pedal, and we were on our way into Vermont. The topography of Vermont consisted of mountains, mountains and more mountains.

When I climbed over the Continental Divide, it seemed like everything else would roll down to the Atlantic. That didn't happen, but none of us were prepared for what we would encounter those last three days.

The staff was aware, but they didn't say much except there would be a little more climbing before we finished. They knew the cyclists didn't want to hear the truth.

As we pedaled out of the parking lot, I didn't need to look for anyone to tag. Gabriel was with me, so I would not be starting the day alone. We were planning to enjoy the day together.

The other cyclists enthusiastically shouted out, "Have a great day!" No one uttered the unsaid words, "Do you think you can waltz out of that van and survive the entire day?"

Gabriel looked like the "stud muffin" of the group with his shiny bronze skin and flexing muscles.

We rolled along the first ten miles at a leisurely pace, enjoying the towering trees and the sparkling water cascading down the hillsides. Gabriel was feeling like a kid, having a ball, and relishing his freedom. He raced ahead; and, true to his word, was waiting for me by one of the shimmering creek pools.

Some of the other riders joined us for a while and then moved on. One of the leaders rode with us for a few miles and then sped away. She had assumed the responsibility to see that Gabriel was okay.

As we started up a long climb, Gabriel and I were chatting away. The further we went, the less talking I heard:

only heavy breathing came out of his mouth. Gabriel had been an asthmatic child and it didn't take much to get him huffing and puffing. Climbing was hard work and conversations naturally dropped off.

Knowing it was going to be a long day, I started creeping ahead of him. When I came to a fork in the road, I did the waiting. Time was ticking away, and that made me nervous. Gabriel finally showed up after fifteen minutes. He was already dragging. He gasped, "I'm fine – let's go."

Up we went. I knew I had to complete the day whether he did or not. I said, "Baby, I can't wait for you again, or I'm not going to make it before dark."

He assured me, "I've gotten my second wind and I'll be right behind you."

As I looked in my tiny rear view mirror, I noticed him disappearing out of sight. It made me sad to pull off and leave him. First of all, I didn't want to hurt his feelings. Secondly, I was worried what might happen to him on the road. He didn't have a clue how careful we had to be to stay alive.

I heard the sag wagon approaching. It pulled over and stopped. So did I. The driver said one of the leaders would be keeping a close eye on Gabriel as she was riding sweep (the back person on the road).

She had made her presence known a few miles back even though she hadn't said what she was doing. That made me feel a little better; it wouldn't salvage Gabriel's pride, but at least someone would be in the rear if he collapsed in a heap alongside the road.

Sometime during the next hour, she pedaled up to me and said, "I found Gabriel hanging on to a bridge railing, hardly able to breathe."

She had called the sag wagon. It happened to be close, turned around and came up beside Gabriel. He pleaded, "Please, give me a lift to the top of the hill, so I can get my reward. I'll be fine after the downhill."

214

Gratefully, he climbed into the sag. He started to get some air back into his lungs as they took off up to the top of the mountain.

There were several of us dawdling on the long climb, so the sweep rode back and forth to check on us.

The next time she went back to check on Gabriel, he was again clinging to a railing and barely breathing. He was inching up the steep incline by pulling himself along the bridge railings. Again the sweep wanted to call the sag and have him picked up but he begged her, "Please, let me try to get up this climb by myself."

He still felt in his heart that he could make the rest of the day, if he could only enjoy the next "downhill" ride. She finally relented. He somehow dragged and pedaled his bike and body up the hill.

Along the way, though, he almost got killed. He was riding in the dreaded clip-on shoes that panic me. He had no choice, as that was what had been left outside our door by a "real biker." Gabriel would never admit he didn't know how to use them. It takes practice to pull your feet off quickly with the half turn of the foot. With no experience, when he tried, one foot got stuck. He toppled over onto the roadway (just like my own experience before I started the ride). When you go over with no forward motion of your bike, you have one leg under the bike with the bike itself and your own body weight pinning you down on the pavement. It takes time to extricate yourself. The truck roaring up the hill missed his head by inches.

He somehow made it to the top and what a reward it was. He tore down that mountainside at breakneck speed, foolishly thinking he was a teenager again. The only problem: that wasn't the last mountain. He started climbing again, but he knew his big ride was over. He clutched the railing, gasping for air. When the sweep found him, he didn't even have enough wind left to argue with her.

Her final admonition was, "You're not going to have a heart attack while I'm on duty. You have to get in the wagon."

He was so close to a complete state of collapse that he slumped into the seat of the wagon without a whimper. They taxied him ahead the next thirty-one miles to the hotel. The way he looked when I found him, someone must have put him on a baggage cart and dumped him on the bed in our room.

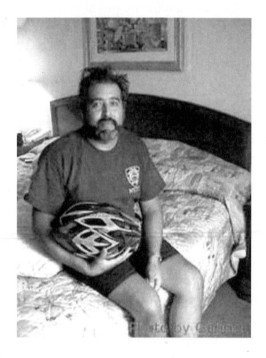

It had looked like a short day on paper, an eighty-one mile day; but the reality was we had climbed 5900 feet.

Gabriel's description of the day in our log was as follows:

"Road kill is not the word for it. When I got picked up, the driver thought I was dead. I climbed one of the toughest days and paid the price. My neck hurts, my BUTT hurts, I have cramps in my legs, arms and feet. I tried to do it all the way,

216

but I guess without the training, it was not a good idea. Patricia and this gang are all awesome!!!!!! Well, I will lie down, as I am still trying to get rid of the stars flashing in my eyes. I will swallow my pride and ride in the van tomorrow."

He had been in the hotel for a few hours by the time I limped in. My leg pain was still excruciating, but it paled in comparison to how much Gabriel was suffering. He started to revive enough to at least walk down for dinner.

By now the word of "mighty Gabriel's ride" had circulated among the cyclists. They were still congratulating and commending him for hanging in there for fifty miles. Not one cyclist said, "I told you so."

Day 49:
Brattleboro, VT to
Manchester, NH

86 miles

May the bicycle Gods have mercy on us. After almost 6,000 feet of climbing yesterday, I was hoping we could coast to the Atlantic. Dream on, Patricia! We had conquered the Green Mountains, but still had to climb the White Mountains. They were all beginning to look alike.

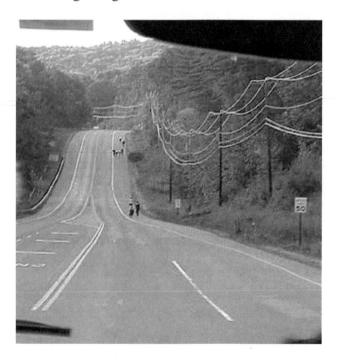

What a magical moment it was when we crossed over into New Hampshire. My dream was almost within reach, if only I could endure the pain.

Medical update:

My leg? I kept waking up during the night and bursting into tears. I was allergic to pain medication, and realized I couldn't be on my bicycle feeling "fuzzy." Gabriel would massage my leg to enable me to get a few winks until the pain jolted me awake again.

The color? If you liked rainbows, my leg was gorgeous: blue, green, purple, pink and every other hue imaginable.

The miracle? There was no swelling. Thank you, guardian angel.

My injured breast? Extremely sore to the touch but not aggravated by cycling.

My mental state? Going forward, regardless of pain.

Comic relief? Thinking of Gabriel yesterday as he lay moaning on our bed. He's not feeling so well either; but at least he's crumpled into a van seat, not on the road pedaling.

When I saw him at the first sag stop, I asked, "How does that nice, soft seat feel in the sag wagon?"

He replied, "It may be soft and upholstered, but all I can feel is the memory of that bicycle seat stuffed up my ass yesterday."

I teased, "I guess some people just aren't tough enough to be cyclists."

The hush-hush about the next-to-last day made me uneasy. We all knew there was climbing on the agenda for today, but no one would tell us what to expect.

We were climbing from the moment we got on our bicycles. The faster, stronger cyclists were leading the pack, but we were only spread over a few miles during the climb. I was surviving; that was all. Next thing I knew, we faced an incline that was between fifteen and nineteen percent.

219

It was inhumane!

Many of the cyclists gave up and started pushing their bicycles up a hill almost too steep for walking. Mike and his sag were parked on top along with the few who had pedaled to the top. They were yelling to those of us still down there, "Come on up!"

"You can do it."

"Don't give up now!"

"You're almost there."

Those of us still trying to make it appreciated the encouragement. That was the steepest climb we'd experienced all across America.

I had to keep trying. The other cyclists knew about my determination to pedal every inch, and I felt all the eyes on me. I could barely push my pedals around once before I had to bail off my bike. The clincher was I could jump off, because I did not have the dreaded clip-on cleats. Most cyclists, who did have clip-ons, had to push their bikes. They would have fallen over before they got their feet out of the lock-in position.

Many cyclists had said I wouldn't be able to make the entire ride without clip-ons. Now I had the advantage.

My "back end buddy, Bill" on the recumbent bike was almost beside me. As I looked over at him, I started screaming, "Oh, my God."

I saw the front end of his bike go up in the air as he flipped over backwards. His bike, with its two wheels, looked like a bucking horse throwing him off.

Several people, who were nearby, ran over to help. He had been thrown out of the bicycle as it flipped. Then the bike continued to slide back down the hill.

Bill was yelling, "Goddamn it, Mike, you didn't have to put us in a position like that. I'm really pissed."

He tried to walk up the incline while three of the guys retrieved his bike and pushed it up the hill.

After all the trials and tribulations of the ride, I was not going to give up. The pain was horrible but I kept inching up, one turn of the pedal; stop and jump off; another turn, stop and jump off. Mike and the gang at the top were all cheering for me when I finally came over the crest of the hill.

The exception: Gabriel.

He was in the sag that had gone ahead. He heard about the horrendous climb from some of the first cyclists and didn't even dare think that I could make it. He was afraid I was going to get knocked out of my dream to pedal every inch. When he heard the incredible news I had pedaled to the top, he was ecstatic. He was shouting "Yahoo" and swinging his fists into the air. His eyes were brimming with tears as he sank back into his seat in the van murmuring, "Thank you God." Only he knew the pain I was suffering because of my injuries.

The rest of the day should have been a breeze. My friend, Judith, stayed back to ride with me. Her husband was a racer and an excellent cyclist, and she tried to keep up with him on many of the days. She was pooped and chose to ride with me instead.

I was hurting so badly that we two brought up the rear and didn't even care how slow we were. We would stop and lay down spread-eagle on the grass whenever we had a chance. It felt so good! I was in heaven having someone with me who didn't want to push. I thought that day would continue happily ever after.

We were the last ones to check in at the last sag stop. Everyone else had gone through hours ago.

Judith said, "Patricia, I don't even know how to tell you, but I am so tired, I am getting in the sag wagon. My day is over. I know you will be alone. I am so sorry but I cannot go on."

I felt like a bomb had been dropped on me. I respected the fact she had "gone as far as she could go."

221

I was alone. I guess that was fitting, on the next-to-last day. I'd been alone so many times and in so many places over those last forty-nine days.

The sag left with Gabriel in it, and I hit the road by myself. Tears are dripping on my computer keyboard as I remember all the emotions that surged through my body and soul.

I had no guidance, as my odometer was still silent. There was no phone reception. I was riding injured and in extreme pain. Gabriel was somewhere up front in a sag. The other sag had gone to help someone else. We had already been climbing all day. There were still twenty-five miles to pedal with no support anywhere.

I could have crawled in the sag and gone with them, but – I had a dream. That dream was getting closer even if it seemed a million miles away.

There was no way to get a feeling for mileage without the odometer. As I rode faster and slower as the terrain dictated, it screwed up all attempts for my mind to make an assessment of where I was. All I could do was keep pedaling. My angel kept me company and calmed my emotions as the miles ticked off. Somehow, I made it to the hotel.

That was the last night for our group to be together. A special dinner and party had been planned. I had to forego the "luxurious" bath and take a quickie shower as I rushed to get ready.

The restaurant was only a few blocks from our hotel. When we got there, they weren't quite ready for us.

As all the cyclists gathered outside, the main chatter concerned the "impossible" climb we had done. Some of the cyclists were really angry that we had such a challenge with only two days to go.

Jonathan said, "What in the hell did Mike think he was doing? There had to be other ways to get here."

Tom spoke up, "I understand Mike is an Olympian."

222

Jim chimed in, "Do you think he was getting his jollies by watching all of us struggle up that ridiculous climb?"

Robert added, "There's no reason to stress everyone out this near the end."

What a party! What an evening! The camaraderie of the group was electric. We had started in Astoria as strangers. Now we were friends with a fabulous feat to share – we had pedaled America. Everyone had their own goal at the start. Thirty-two had gone all across country. Thirteen or fourteen of us had actually pedaled all the miles. The others had taken time out when they needed it, either for fatigue or injuries. I knew my goal of pedaling every inch would be decided tomorrow. With the help of my angel, I would succeed.

After dinner, we all enjoyed a combination of skits, jokes, and whatever anyone wanted to contribute. Each of us had an opportunity to speak when we were presented with our engraved certificate of completion.

When it was my turn, I finished with, "I'm probably the most unlikely cyclist you've ever had in my Hanes hose, short shorts and no clip-ons. I'll be remembered as the most "unbicyclist" bicycle rider to ever pedal across America."

We still had to pedal into Portsmouth the next day but ABB must have had confidence in us as our certificates were signed.

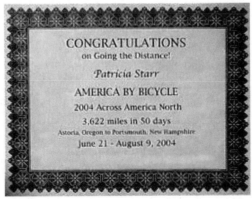

CONGRATULATIONS
on Going the Distance!

Patricia Starr

AMERICA BY BICYCLE

2004 Across America North

3,622 miles in 50 days

Astoria, Oregon to Portsmouth, New Hampshire

June 21 - August 9, 2004

Day 50:
Manchester, NH to
Portsmouth, NH

60 miles

I did it again—I felt those tears slipping out from under my glasses. After all those long days on the road and the obstacles I had overcome – ominous electrical storms, rain, heat, wind, fatigue, hunger, traffic, a broken toe, muscles screaming at me from my encounter with the bridge railing, panic at being lost and alone, enduring the mental hardship of losing our van and possessions, dealing with an alcoholic husband----was my dream of reaching the Atlantic going to be thwarted on the last day by a broken bicycle chain?

Electricity was in the air from the moment I woke up. Was the day really here? The day I had dreamed about for a year and a half?

The last four days were "mind over matter." My throbbing leg had kept me awake again last night. I would have to endure pain to finish the ride and accomplish my dream.

Everyone was on a real high that morning at breakfast. We had to ride 48 miles by 11:00 a.m. and then find our way to the Junior High School where a police escort would pick us up at 11:30. They would lead us *en masse* to the Atlantic Ocean to dip our front tires in the water.

Fifty days ago we had dipped the rear tires in the Pacific Ocean. The symbolism of "coast to coast" was about to take place. The excitement of the coming moment was unbearable. Was the 67 year old broad in Hanes Pantyhose going to be able to say she had pedaled across America – every inch of it?

I knew I would be pedaling frantically to reach the destination on time. We were in New Hampshire; and although we wouldn't have the climbing we had conquered and endured the past two days, it didn't look like the flats of Wyoming.

My stomach felt like butterflies were jumping around in it as I slipped onto my bicycle and found someone I could tag out of the parking lot – an important step even on the last day.

We lucked out again; the weather was cool and the scenery was breathtaking with towering pine trees everywhere.

After being on the road for fifty days, I felt like I was in great shape except for injuries. Everyone else was too, though, so I was still working like crazy to keep up with the pack. I had lost seven or eight pounds even though I ate constantly. The amount of calories it took to ride America was astronomical. Actually, I was too skinny – my ribs showed when I stretched. Most of America probably wished for my problem!

We stayed close for the first half hour. Then the faster riders began to pull away. Some still had the goal of being the first to arrive after all of those miles on the road. I had been so thankful each day "to arrive." We were really cruising, and I was struggling. Oh-oh – a long, steep climb – they never did tell us everything at breakfast.

The first one went without incident, although many of the pack passed me. I wished I had a light bike and a granny gear. I should have thought of that before I started in Astoria, but how could I have known the reality of the road.

Only a few of us remained to conquer the next mountain. As I was pushing really hard on the pedals, I heard an ominous clink and crack sound coming from my chain. It froze completely and would not turn the pedals. I picked up my bike and hurried off the roadway to investigate. No one stopped, as we all had the same objective, to get there.

As several passed by, they yelled, "Are you OK?"

225

I yelled back, "I don't think so. My chain was making a horrible, grinding noise and isn't turning."

Someone yelled back, "It's probably slipping gears." (In other words, it was broken).

My heart sank. I had seen other bikers "trapped" on the roadside from the same malady. All you could do was wait for the repair wagon and hope they weren't ahead of you. With my slow pace, they were always ahead.

A chain could be replaced. The problem was Mike, the ABB leader, had stressed many times at breakfast that the procession to the beach would leave at 11:30 sharp. We had better be there, because it would wait for no one. Was I going to be the one denied the final opportunity to celebrate with the entire pack after all those days on the road—3,622 miles?

The other problem was my non-functioning odometer – that was the third day I couldn't even get a peep out of it no matter how many buttons I pushed. I was alone *again* with no mileage information to help me find my way on the map.

I also didn't know what time it was, which was probably a good thing, or there would have been more knots in my stomach. I couldn't see what was causing my bike to be non-functioning; but I turned it upside down so if anyone was on the road behind me, they would know I was in serious trouble.

After all of those days, my guardian angel had not abandoned me. When I turned my bike upside down, a stone that had been lodged between the teeth and the chain flipped out. I grabbed the pedals with my hands and the miracle happened – they turned freely. I jumped up and down and yelled "Thank you God" at the top of my lungs in the lush, lonely forest.

Tears spilled down my checks onto my ABB jersey with all the stars on it. Nothing was going to stop me now. The only thing I didn't know was the time factor. Was I going to get to the church (school) on time?

After pedaling about ten miles, I was getting a little uneasy. There should have been a sag wagon or the sweep on the road somewhere. I checked my map and realized there was an unmarked turn to the right that only could have been correctly measured by having a working odometer.

Now what do I do? Keep riding forward? Turn around to go back? Risk losing road time and miss the procession to the beach?

I started to panic. I couldn't handle any more obstacles. It wasn't fair. As I was trying to figure out what to do, I saw two bicyclists in the distance. I jumped off my bike and waved at them. When they got close, I yelled, "Please help me – I'm lost."

They yelled back, "So are we!" One of the men had been riding with the group on part of the ride. The other rider was his brother who had "come along for the ride" into Portsmouth, so he couldn't be of any help.

We tried to figure out what to do. We decided to keep riding to see if we could find a house, a car or a person. After a few miles, we saw a car coming toward us. We flagged it down and a nice, pretty lady said she was a visitor and couldn't make any sense out of our map. There went another hope dashed onto the pavement.

What now? We got back on our bikes and continued down the road. We didn't have a clue what we were doing. But it felt like we were doing something if we were on our bikes and pedaling. After another couple of miles, we saw a pickup truck approaching. We jumped off our bikes and flagged him down.

As the words tumbled out of our mouths that we were lost and had to get to the school outside of Portsmouth by 11:30, he studied our direction sheet. He said, "Continue ahead for two miles until you see a fork in the road. Take the left fork and it will put you on a back way leading into town."

The other alternative was to turn around and go back almost seven miles to find the unmarked right turn that we had missed. That option would surely make us late for the procession to the beach.

We thanked him profusely, jumped on our bikes and raced down the road. After a couple of miles, we saw the fork in the road as promised. Nothing could stop us now.

I was pedaling like crazy to keep up with the two experienced bicyclists. After a few miles, there it was, straight ahead, the familiar and dreaded signs we had seen all across America – DETOUR AHEAD – BRIDGE OUT – with signs pointing to the left. That couldn't be happening to us. It was our last day and we were not going to make it by 11:30 if we had to detour. We knew from experience that detours in the country could be from four to ten extra miles. It was not like being in the city and going around the block. That didn't even factor in the extra climbs we'd have to deal with.

The other two cyclists wanted to try for the detour. I was afraid we would be late, so I spoke up. "Let's just ignore the signs and go for it. Sometimes, when the bridges are out, there might be a little trail to follow from side to side if it was not over a big, rushing stream."

I wasn't usually so forceful; but the other two realized I was dead serious, so they said, "Okay, let's go for it."

At least the Russian roulette gamble gave us a chance.

My angel came to the rescue again. As we approached the construction mess ahead, we saw that the bridge had been completely disassembled. However, there was a tiny walkway over the abyss leading to the other side. The catwalk was only a couple of feet wide, accessible for a person to walk, but we had to walk and push a bicycle beside us.

"Oh my God," I moaned. "I can't step out on that sliver of a board, and with my bike beside me? No way!"

My mind instantly flipped back to my childhood in the cornfields of Nebraska. As farmers who had barely survived

228

the dust bowl, the only real entertainment we had was a yearly trip to Lincoln, thirty miles away, to see the circus when it came to town. Somehow, my folks managed to afford the tickets for the annual extravaganza. The aerialists and their feats way up at the top of the tent mesmerized me. I can still remember how constricted my chest felt, as I held my breath while they teetered across the tiny wire so high in the air. Was I expected to do the same feat?

The other cyclists said, "Come on, Patricia. It was your idea to come this way. Are you chickening out now? The last day?"

I meekly replied, "No."

It was no time to be afraid of heights. We slowly stepped out, one by one, with our bicycles at our sides, and made it across to the other side. And, yes, my chest was hurting; some memories last forever.

Thank you, guardian angel. My decision had been the right one. As we cleared the construction site, we noticed a car parked by the road. We jumped off our bikes and ran over to the driver. "Please, where are we?"

She said, "You're less than five miles from town."

Her answer was greeted by war whoops from all three of us.

No one could have envisioned the agony and the ecstasy that extended even into the last day. I knew how close I was to achieving the dream of riding America, and still it seemed like I was never going to get there.

As we rode into town, I felt like my heart was going to race right out of my body. We pedaled down the street to the junior high. Then all the red, white, and blue bicycle shirts dotted with stars came into view. The police cars were lined up ready for the procession, and everyone was standing around chatting and laughing. I had been dreaming about that moment for fifty days.

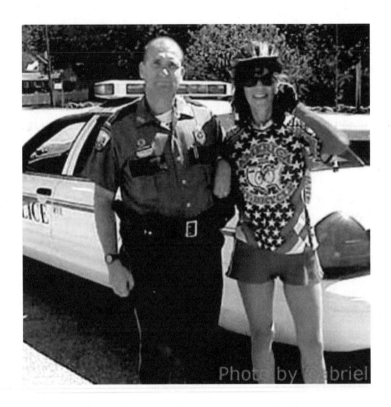

Before we took off for the historic procession to the beach, everyone gathered on the steps of the school for group pictures. It was so easy to put a big smile on my face.

Gabriel grabbed his movie camera bag to record the awesome day. When I looked out at the crowd gathered around us, I saw him frantically waving a little red, tattered book. Happiness tears spilled out of my eyes. The book he was waving was something my mother made for me that I thought was gone forever.

When our van was stolen and burned one week ago in Brantford, Canada, I agonized about our earthly possessions that had been so brutally and senselessly destroyed. The one item that could not be replaced was my address book.

In the Santa Barbara inferno of 1977 called the Sycamore Fire, every earthly possession was incinerated in thirty seconds when our house exploded from the intense heat. A few weeks later, the book came in the mail from my mom in Omaha, Nebraska. She had compiled all the addresses of our family and hand-written them in the book.

The trauma of losing every visible item of my past was hard enough to endure. The feeling I had lost touch with every person in my family was unbearable.

My mother took care of that. The little red book was my treasure and my only link to the past. It was tattered and torn and the pages were falling out, but I never once entertained the thought of writing it over in my handwriting or putting the information in my computer.

It had even more meaning because it was in my mother's handwriting. When she died at age 90, her handwriting was still the same distinct round shaped letters she had learned to do in a little country school in Nebraska.

I would never have left home on the fabulous adventure of riding America without that book. The assumption that it had disappeared in another horrible inferno had broken my heart.

But somehow the book had found its way into Gabriel's movie camera bag. Neither of us knew how it got there or why it was there. After the destruction of the van, the only possessions he had were the ones he had taken into the hotel room in Brantford – the movie camera bag, his computer, and the clothes on his back. Now, as I stood on the steps with the rest of the gang that had shared the awesome experience, I looked out into the crowd and saw my husband running back and forth waving the little red address book.

The address book in my mother's distinctive handwriting was a survivor – like the feeling going through my body at that moment. No matter what had transpired on those long, long fifty days, I too was a survivor.

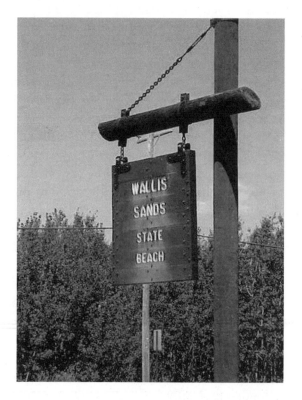

The entourage took off on the long-awaited ride to the beach. Two patrol cars led us. A third car brought up the rear. It was exciting to be riding as a group. We had only done that once before when the bridge from Port Huron to Canada was closed so we could all ride over together, undisturbed by the normal traffic.

Gabriel had grabbed the extra bike from the ABB van. He had no intention of missing those moments, so he was riding with no hands – both of his hands were steadying his movie camera. He was leading the pack of riders and weaving back and forth to get as much footage as possible. He had spent fifty days being the ultimate PR man, and he needed some concluding shots.

The ABB director was perturbed because Gabriel was not setting a good riding example. But, it worked, and he got what he needed.

As we neared the beach, Gabriel got another reward. All his diligence to keep me in the eye of the media had paid off. The local camera crew from Portsmouth was there at the beach to greet me. We needed all the publicity we could get as we still had many dollars to raise to fund the Patricia Starr Music Scholarship at Santa Barbara City College.

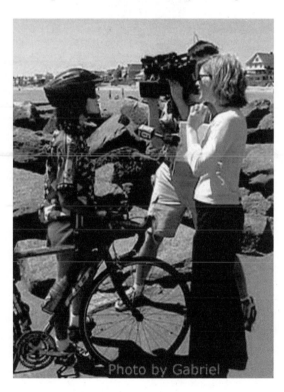

Photo by Gabriel

As I dipped my front wheel in the Atlantic Ocean, the TV station recorded it and interviewed me. Then my angel worked one more little miracle. Unbeknown to us, the local TV station was an ABC affiliate that was happy to share the information. I dunked my tire at 2:00 p.m. and they fired it back to our local station KEYT-3. John Palminteri had it on local Santa Barbara News at 5:00 p.m. that afternoon.

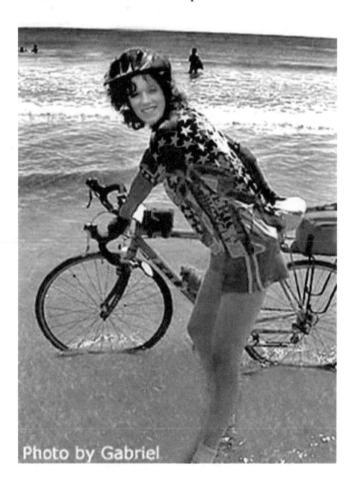

Photo by Gabriel

The emotional moment was absolutely overwhelming. Of course I was crying; but that time it wasn't loneliness, fear, hunger, heat, frustration, or pain. What a glorious feeling to know I had overcome every obstacle put in front of me. I had survived. I had accomplished something spectacular most people only dream about. In doing so, I was funding a scholarship that will be in perpetuity for music majors at our local college.

I, Patricia Starr, at age 67, had pedaled my bicycle all the way across America—3,622 miles from Astoria, Oregon to Portsmouth, New Hampshire.

"To achieve all that is possible,
you must attempt the impossible.
To be as much as you can be,
you must dream of being more.
Your dream is the promise of ALL you can be."
(Author unknown)

235

CREDITS

To Tom Locashio, our computer guru and long-time friend who made the website and kept it current with daily updates: You had many fans across the country as they waited every day to see how Patricia was handling all the challenges and if she was still alive! Your expertise and ingenuity made this fun and informative for everyone. Your magic with graphics enhances "Angel" and adds a new dimension for the reader.

To Jolinda Newton Pizzirani, our publisher, we are so grateful for your knowledge, guidance and caring to make "Angel" a success. We knew we were in good hands from the moment you offered to bring this part of our dream to fruition. We are thrilled to be another of your angel success stories!

To husband Gabriel, all of your gorgeous photographs have helped to bring "Angel" alive to all of our readers. Your discriminating "eye" to catch the moment encourages the reader to be right there on the road--both suffering and enjoying with Patricia as she survives each day.

To the Baron, radio 1290, for his continued encouragement before, during and after the ride with in studio interviews and daily contact across America. His loyal listeners and all of his "Lunch Bunch" groupies were the support that made my wings fly.

And to every contributor to the Patricia Starr Scholarship Fund at Santa Barbara City College, we say thank you--from large donations and support from Silvio and Mary DiLoreto to children's donations of nickels and pennies. The $22,000 was raised and the $1,000 a year scholarship is now in perpetuity.

Also Available From
Summerland Publishing

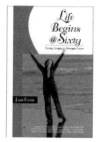

"Life Begins@Sixty" by Joan Frentz. "The strength of this book lies in relating to the kind of deep-down feelings and challenges we women face every day: taking up the treadmill yet another time or eating a decadent hunk of chocolate because there was no hope. It was comforting to know that I am not alone. "Life Begins@Sixty" is not just for women over sixty. It's for every woman who has bought new clothes because the old didn't fit any longer. It's for every woman who has been on every single diet on earth. It's for every woman who knows she has to get out there and start living better but just hasn't been able to." - Magai Pitchai, Literary Editor

US$15.95/CAN$20.95   ISBN: 978-0-9794863-4-0

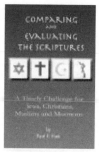

That religions profoundly affect our lives in innumerable ways, no one is likely to dispute. Disagreements emerge, however, when we attempt to evaluate those effects, and when we attempt to determine religion's proper place in our lives, in our society, and in our troubled world. Wouldn't it be worthwhile for everyone to think through our religious traditions one more time, from the beginning? Isn't it possible to resolve some of the issues involved in a manner that is less militant and more intelligent? **"Comparing and Evaluating the Scriptures"** by Paul Fink will give readers the opportunities they seek to develop clear answers to these questions are and? more.

US16.95 / CAN $21.95   ISBN: 978-0-9795444-3-9

Order from:
www.summerlandpublishing.com,
www.barnesandnoble.com, www.amazon.com
or find it in your favorite bookstore!
Email Info@SummerlandPublishing.com
for more information.

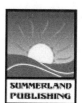

Summerland Publishing, 21 Oxford Drive, Lompoc, CA 93436

Angel On My Handlebars
printed on

Recycled paper
"Doing my part"

DISCARD